Keto Friendly Recipes

~~~

EASY
KETO
FOR BUSY
PEOPLE

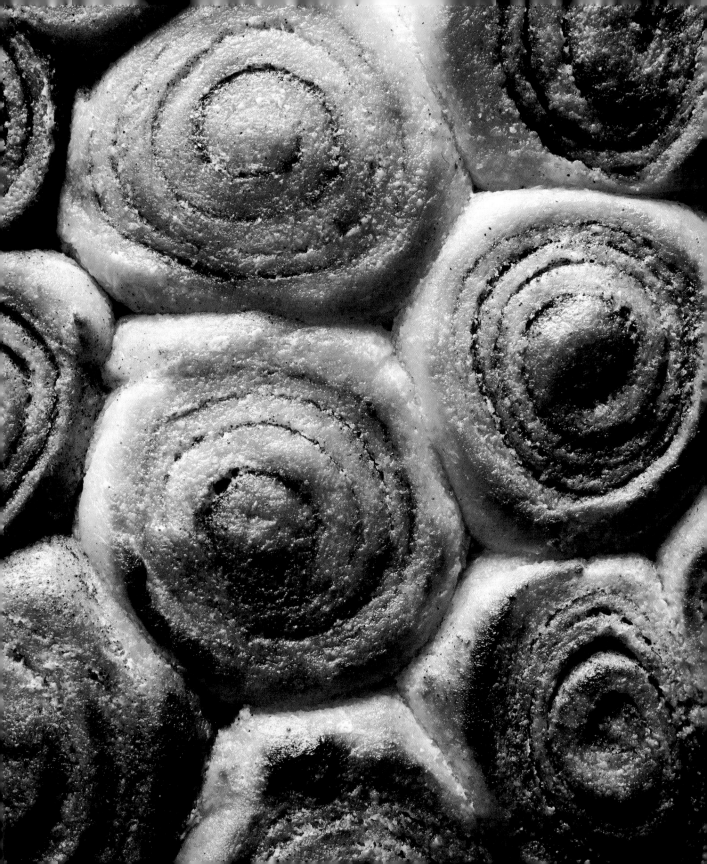

Keto Friendly Recipes

〜

EASY KETO FOR BUSY PEOPLE

〜

JENNIFER MARIE GARZA

Photography by Ghazalle Badiozamani

HOUGHTON MIFFLIN HARCOURT
BOSTON NEW YORK 2019

Copyright © 2019 by Jennifer Marie Garza
Photography copyright © 2019 by Ghazalle Badiozamani
Food styling by Barrett Washburne
Prop styling by Jenna Tedesco

All rights reserved.
For information about permission to reproduce selections from this book, write
to trade.permissions@hmhco.com or to Permissions, Houghton Mifflin Harcourt
Publishing Company, 3 Park Avenue, 19th Floor, New York, New York 10016.
hmhbooks.com

Library of Congress Cataloging-in-Publication Data
Names: Garza, Jennifer Marie, author.
Title: Keto friendly recipes : easy keto for busy people / Jennifer Marie Garza.
Description: Boston : Houghton Mifflin Harcourt, 2019. | Includes index.
Identifiers: LCCN 2019001732 (print) | LCCN 2019004692 (ebook) |
ISBN 9780358123026 (ebook) | ISBN 9780358120865 (paperback) |
ISBN 9780358123026 (ebk)
Subjects: LCSH: Low-carbohydrate diet—Recipes. | BISAC: COOKING /
Health & Healing / Low Carbohydrate. | COOKING / Health & Healing /
Weight Control. | HEALTH & FITNESS / Weight Loss. | LCGFT: Cookbooks.
Classification: LCC RM237.73 (ebook) | LCC RM237.73 .G374 2019 (print) |
DDC 641.5/6383—dc23
LC record available at https://lccn.loc.gov/2019001732

Book design by Allison Chi

Printed in the United States of America
DOC 10 9 8 7 6 5 4 3 2 1

To my husband, John, who always has my six no matter how crazy my ideas are. I love you! To my daughters, Megan and Melanie, you are my everything.

CONTENTS

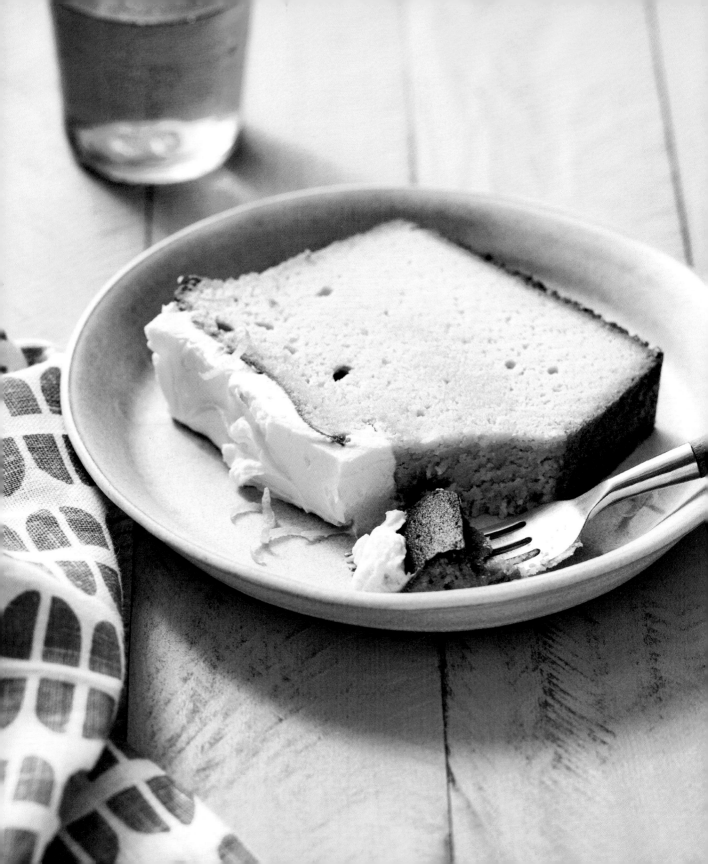

ACKNOWLEDGMENTS

To my editor, Justin Schwartz, thank you for believing in me. Your hard work and expertise on this project have taught me so much, and I am very happy I had the opportunity to work with you on it.

To my agent, Lisa Grubka, thank you for helping me and giving me your valuable advice.

To Amy Treadwell, a huge thank-you to you for helping me express exactly what I was trying to say. I could not have done this without you.

Special thanks to Ghazalle Badiozamani for photography, Barrett Washburne for food styling, and Jenna Tedesco for prop styling. Your talents are remarkable and I am glad to have you all on my team!

To my family—my husband, John, and my beautiful daughters, Megan and Melanie—I am so thankful that you have supported me in my dream to create this cookbook. I could not have done this without all of your ideas, recipe testing, and the chores you took over to take some of the work off my hands. Thank you for always supporting me in everything I do!

To my mom, dad, and brother, Raymond, thank you for your love and support.

To my friend Andrea Deckard, thank you for being my confidante, cheerleader, and sounding board. I am forever grateful for your friendship and guidance.

To all of my blogger friends and secret mastermind partners, thank you! I would not be where I am today without you. I value your friendship more than you will ever know.

To Dr. Annette Bosworth, thank you for helping me understand the science behind my own weight-loss journey as I have followed the ketogenic diet. I am grateful for your friendship.

To the members of the Low Carb Inspirations group on Facebook, thank you for being part of an online community that has helped me through my own journey. I hope to return the positivity tenfold. Special thanks to Becky Grimmer, Michelle Ierna, and Kris Dee for helping to moderate such a positive group of low-carb and keto people! You gals are the best!

To the members of the Beef and Butter Fast 5-Day Challenge Facebook group, thank you for trusting me and my crazy process to help you get out of a keto weight-loss stall. I always look forward to our monthly challenges.

And last but not least, thank you to everyone who follows my blogging adventures online. Your comments and questions keep my desire going! I am forever grateful.

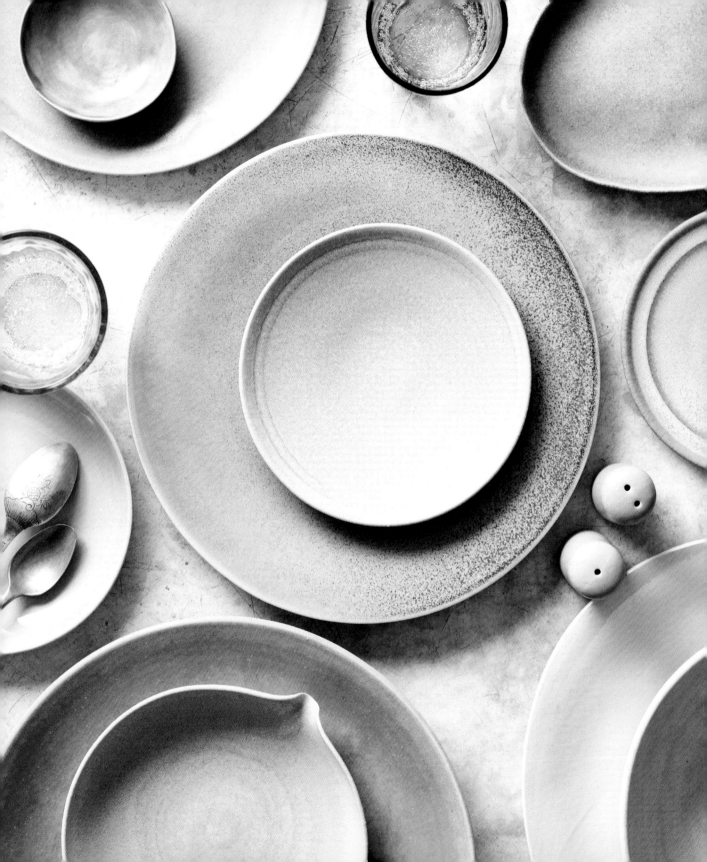

INTRODUCTION

MY KETO STORY

I've always struggled with my weight. Carbohydrates and sugar controlled my life for far too long. I tried every diet on the planet only to fail with every attempt. I thought I just didn't have the willpower that others had. Plus, my blood sugar would not allow me to go hungry for very long without feeling unwell, and that made dieting even harder.

When I heard about the keto way of life and its ability to help with weight loss, I was intrigued and decided to give it a go. I vividly remember the day—January 27, 2017—that I cleaned out my pantry of all the foods I was used to consuming but that no longer fit into my newfound keto diet.

Two weeks later, I was holding strong to my weight loss goals, and my husband asked where I wanted to eat on Valentine's Day. I was worried that if we went to a restaurant, I'd end up eating the wrong foods, either because they were too tempting or without realizing it (restaurants don't tell you every ingredient that goes into a dish), so I suggested we buy some rib eye steaks and celebrate at home instead. It was right then and there that we both realized I was serious about this new way of eating.

Fortunately, just because I was on the keto diet did not mean I had to deprive myself of food that tasted great. I was determined to make delicious meals that not only conformed to the diet requirements, but that my family would also love. I didn't want any of us to think of this way of eating as a restrictive diet, and once I understood the basic rules, I knew that keto was much more than that. It was a way of eating that anyone could make a part of their lives.

Embarking on a new healthy lifestyle can be intimidating and scary, especially when you're just beginning and don't have all the answers and are inundated by information. But don't let that stop you from starting the diet. If I can do it, so can you!

Today, I have lost 55 pounds and I feel wonderful. I have never stayed with a diet plan this long, ever, and I think it's because it's not very hard to follow and I actually like to eat the food. Carbs and sugar no longer have a hold on me like they did. I may have started this plan to lose weight, but now it's simply the way I live every day, and the way my family lives too. It's amazing that small, simple changes in your food choices can change your whole life. Not only has this helped my waistline, but I feel better and have so much energy.

I decided to write this book because it's become my life's mission to share the knowledge I have gained and my love for creating recipes to help others who have struggled like I have. I found that you don't need to eat crazy, unheard-of ingredients that you can't pronounce (let alone find at the grocery store), and you don't need to spend a ton of time in the kitchen either. In my mind, a diet will never work unless the food tastes wonderful and doesn't leave you feeling as though you've missed out on anything. That's exactly what I'm giving you with the recipes in this book. Good food that tastes great!

THE KETO DIET

There are two ways our bodies can burn fuel. We can burn ketones, or we can burn glucose. The goal of the keto diet is to get your body burning ketones—to get into ketosis. Keto is a low-carbohydrate, high-fat, moderate-protein diet based on your body's macronutrient needs. Typically, the ratio is 75 percent fat, 20 percent protein, and 5 percent carbs. When your body switches into ketosis, it burns fat as its main fuel source. When you restrict carbohydrates, sugar, and monounsaturated fats, your body will go into ketosis and start burning fat instead of storing it. Most people eat carbohydrates as their main fuel source and burn glucose (sugar). But if you burn fat as your main source of fuel, you won't feel hunger so quickly—and you'll start to lose

weight. I promise, this is the reason I have been able to do this diet successfully. (Note: When your body consumes more protein than it needs, it can turn that excess into glucose which is a process known as gluconeogenesis, and this will interfere with weight loss. That's why it's important to eat the right proportions of fat, carbs, and protein.)

The following will give you more information about ketones and how to calculate your own macronutrients based on your body fat, activity level, and weight.

Types of Ketones

When you burn fat, your body produces ketones. There are three different types of ketones:

1. Beta-hydroxybutyrate, which is found in the blood.
2. Acetoacetate, which is found in the urine.
3. Acetone, which is found in the breath.

There are three different ways to test to see if you are in ketosis. This is important to track because once you are in ketosis, your body will be working as efficiently as possible, which will promote weight loss.

1. Blood meter: Measures the amount of beta-hydroxybutyrate and is the most accurate form of testing.
2. Urine strips: These measure acetoacetate in your urine. The strips can be helpful in the beginning of your journey but will eventually give you a false reading as you utilize the ketones in your body after you become fat-adapted.

BEFORE

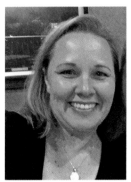 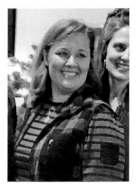

"I may have started this plan to lose weight, but now it's simply the way I live every day."

AFTER

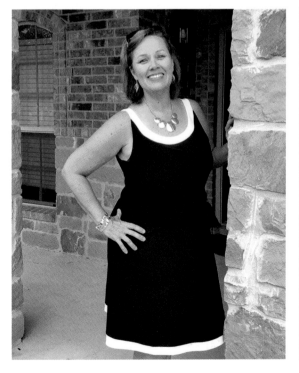 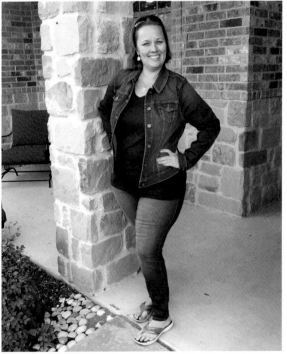

3. Ketone breathalyzer: Acetone can be read by these devices, which provide an accurate and noninvasive tool for measuring acetone in your breath.

You can purchase a blood meter and urine strips at your local Walmart or drugstore. All three items are available to purchase online on Amazon.

Macronutrients

Macronutrients consist of fats, protein, and carbs. There are two factors that influence your macronutrient levels: activity level and lean mass weight. It's important to maintain your body's correct macronutrient ratio to get into ketosis, so it switches your body's fuel source from glucose to ketones.

You can find out what your specific macronutrient needs are by using a macronutrient calculator, which you can find online by searching for *keto macronutrient calculator.* There are many to choose from, and most are easy to use. Try a couple to find the one that feels right for you.

The calculator will determine the exact amount of macronutrients you need to consume in order to achieve ketosis. Most calculators will ask for the following information, though this may vary from calculator to calculator:

- Gender
- Age
- Height
- Weight
- Activity Level
- Body Fat Percentage

Here's an example of how they work:

First you need to figure out your body fat percentage. To determine your body fat, you will need a DEXA scan, which is available at gyms, or by request at some doctors' offices.

Your lean mass weight is your weight in pounds minus the weight of your body fat. For example, if you weigh 160 pounds and your DEXA scan says you have 30 percent body fat, your lean mass weight would be 112 pounds. ($160 - 30\% = 112$ pounds.)

Multiply the result by 0.6 (grams of protein per pound of lean body mass—that is your target goal) to determine the minimum grams of protein you should consume each day. Therefore, $112 \text{ pounds} \times 0.6 = 67$ grams of protein, the minimum you should consume on a daily basis. You should never consume more grams of protein than the number of your lean mass weight.

In this example, the minimum amount of protein you should consume is 67 grams, but you should not go over 112 grams of protein in a day.

Activity Levels

Use these basic guidelines to determine your own activity level.

SEDENTARY: Very little or no exercise at all.
LIGHTLY ACTIVE: Light exercise such as walking or cycling one to three times a week.
MODERATELY ACTIVE: Moderate cardio or muscle training three to five times a week.
VERY ACTIVE: Hard exercise, muscle training, and/or intense cardio five or more times a week.

ATHLETIC OR BODYBUILDING: High-intensity exercise at a professional level done daily.

Fat Adapted

Being fat adapted means your body is using fat as fuel; it's basically another way to say that you are in ketosis. Fat adaptation implies you have restricted carbs enough to induce and increase the fat-burning process. Once you are fully fat adapted and using fat for your fuel, you are officially in nutritional ketosis. This can take anywhere from a couple of weeks to two months to shift over. Once you become fat-adapted you will probably feel a burst of energy! I remember feeling as though I could run a marathon when my body first moved into ketosis.

Keto Benefits

When you start the keto diet, you will quickly notice the positive attributes that have made this lifestyle so popular.

REDUCED APPETITE

Fat tends to keep you full for a longer time than sugar and carbs. Consuming 75 percent fat in your diet leads to reduced appetite and fewer cravings. You will no longer be controlled by the typical hunger pangs or sugar cravings that occur on other diet plans. With a reduced appetite, you will easily consume fewer calories and that leads to weight loss.

FEWER CRAVINGS

It takes about three days to fully detox your system from the cravings you get from sugar and carbohydrates. Three very rough days. Once that is over, your cravings will be gone! Knowing this in the beginning really helped get me through those first tough days. And I didn't believe I could do it until I actually went through it. I was the most sugar-addicted person on the planet, so if I can get through three days of intense cravings, you can too.

WEIGHT LOSS

The keto diet is also known as a flushing diet. It helps reduce inflammation, which releases water. I vividly remember losing a pound a day for the first eight days following the diet. Rapid weight loss in the beginning is fairly normal. Just remember to supplement with additional electrolytes so you don't get dehydrated.

LOTS OF FAT

It's very important to understand from the beginning that healthy fats are good for you. In the past 20 years we've been taught that fat is bad, when in reality it's the carbs and sugar that are the real culprit. Don't eat anything that says low-fat, fat-free, or reduced-fat! Eating a ketogenic diet of 75 percent fats, 20 percent protein, and only 5 percent carbs will also raise your HDL (good) cholesterol and decrease your triglycerides.

REDUCED RISK FOR DISEASE

You will reduce your risk of high blood pressure, high blood sugar, and diabetes when you reduce the amount of carbohydrates and sugar in your diet.

IMPROVED GUT HEALTH

Sugar, processed foods, and carbohydrates cause inflammation in your intestinal tract. Reducing these in your diet will help foster a healthy gut.

IMPROVED FOCUS AND MENTAL CLARITY

A few weeks into your new keto lifestyle, suddenly you will realize you have improved focus and mental clarity. This really happened to me, and I never realized I was experiencing brain fog until it lifted.

Why You Should Start the Keto Diet

I believe everyone should begin a keto diet or some alternate form of low-carbohydrate plan. The foods available to us today are loaded with so much sugar, it's unbelievable. And I don't think cutting carbs and sugar is beneficial just for weight loss either. I have seen big changes in my kids when I restricted the amount of sugar in their diets. They have better focus, they concentrate more, and they are happier and less irritable. It's absolutely amazing what can happen to your body when you eat real food!

Keto Approved Foods

There are so many delicious foods that can be eaten on the keto diet—many more than the foods you can't. This is one of the

reasons I like this diet so much—I never feel deprived.

What Not to Eat

- Grains: Avoid all grains.
- Fruits: Fruit has tons of sugar. Stick to berries such as strawberries, blueberries, and raspberries, but consume them in small quantities.
- Processed foods: Stay away from anything that has been processed. Stick to fresh "real" foods.
- Root vegetables: Avoid carrots, potatoes, parsnips, rutabagas, and turnips.
- Dairy: Avoid all reduced-fat products.
- Oils: Avoid canola oil, vegetable oil, safflower oil, margarine, Crisco, and hydrogenated cooking oils.
- Sugar and low- or no-calorie sweeteners: Avoid sweeteners such as aspartame and sucralose.
- Cured meats: Avoid all cured deli meats, cured hot dogs, cured bacon, or nitrates in meats.

What to Eat

- Avocado
- Butter
- Cheese
- Coconut aminos
- Coconut vinegar
- Cruciferous vegetables
- Dairy
- Eggs
- Extracts for flavoring
- Fatty cuts of meat

- Ghee
- Greens
- Guar gum or xanthan gum, as a thickening agent
- Heavy cream
- Hot sauce
- Liquid smoke
- MCT oil
- Miracle noodles
- Nut butters such as almond, sunflower, peanut, cashew
- Pepperoni
- Pork rinds
- Protein powders
- Salt
- Squash

Keto Approved Sweeteners

STEVIA GLYCERITE (LIQUID)

- 0 calories
- 300 percent sweeter than sugar
- Conversion: 1 cup sugar = 1 teaspoon stevia

Stevia doesn't affect the blood sugar and has no calories, which helps with weight loss.

ERYTHRITOL (POWDER)

- 0 to 0.2 calories per gram
- 70 percent as sweet as sugar
- Conversion: 1 cup sugar = 1 cup erythritol

If using amounts over 1 cup, I usually add 1 teaspoon stevia glycerite for every 1 cup erythritol to reach a sweetness equal to sugar. For amounts less than 1 cup, you won't notice any difference in sweetness. Erythritol crystallizes and is very similar to sugar. It's

perfect for baking and does not affect blood glucose levels.

MONKFRUIT SWEETENER

- 0 to 0.2 calories per gram
- 100 percent as sweet as sugar
- Conversion: 1 cup sugar = 1 cup monkfruit sweetener

Monkfruit crystallizes and is very similar to sugar. It's also a zero glycemic sweetener that is perfect for baking.

PYURE GRANULATED STEVIA

- 0 to 0.2 calories per gram
- 100 percent as sweet as sugar
- Conversion: 1 cup sugar = 1 cup Pyure

YACON SYRUP (LIQUID)

- 1.5 calories per gram
- 50 percent as sweet as sugar
- Conversion: 1 cup sugar = 2 cups yacon syrup

Yacon syrup is a low-glycemic sweetener that is pressed from the yacon root. It's similar to the consistency of molasses and perfect for baking! It can replace molasses, honey, agave, and maple syrup. I purchase yacon syrup from Amazon.com, though most natural food stores will carry it.

XYLITOL (GRANULATED)

- 2.4 calories per gram
- 100 percent as sweet as sugar
- Conversion: 1 cup sugar = 1 cup xylitol

Xylitol is a naturally occurring alcohol found in most plant material, including many fruits

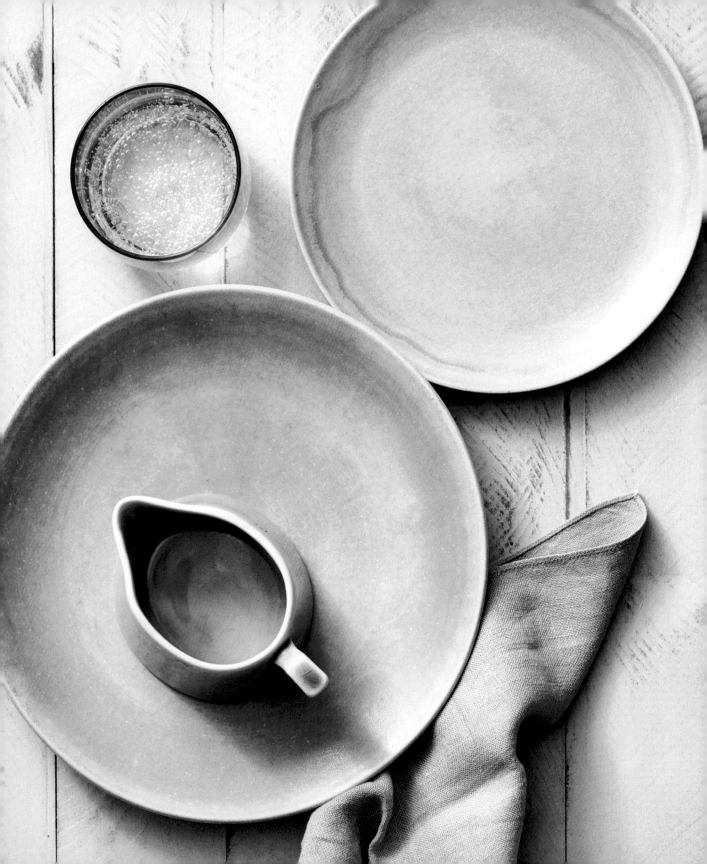

and vegetables. Warning: It is extremely toxic to dogs.

Keto Pantry and Fridge Items

Having the right foods in your pantry will make it much easier to stay on the diet. Knowing sources for the right foods is just as important. Proteins, healthy fats, and vegetables can be found at nearly any local grocery store, but keto snack items might be a bit harder to find.

I tend to shop at Walmart, Costco, Target, H-E-B, Sprouts, and Whole Foods, among others. I've found multiple items on Amazon too. You can find a list of my favorite keto products at bit.ly/KetoFavorites.

HEALTHY FATS

Healthy fats are extremely important on the ketogenic diet. There are good fats and not so good fats.

GOOD FATS: butter, cream, lard, red meat, coconut oil, eggs, palm oil, avocados, avocado oil, cocoa butter, olive oil, macadamia nut oil, goose fat, bacon fat, flaxseed oil, walnuts, fish oil, sesame oil, chia seeds, nut oils.

BAD FATS: Stay away from unhealthy processed trans fats and polyunsaturated fats such as hydrogenated oils, processed vegetable oils, and canola oil.

KETO FLU

When you rid your body of sugar and carbs, you may start to experience what we call the Keto Flu. This is simply your body going through a metabolic change. You might notice a slight headache or even feel nauseated. Other symptoms of Keto Flu could include muscle twitching or cramps, which are signs of low magnesium, which is a common problem. There are things you can do to help. The best thing to do is avoid dehydration by finding a good sugar-free electrolyte supplement. Drink pickle juice (yes, really!) for immediate relief. You can also drink Powerade Zero as needed. Keto Flu symptoms should dissipate after a few days. Another tip is to consume pink Himalayan rock salt, which will provide the minerals you need and help you retain some of the water you are losing. I carry this salt with me when I'm on the go.

APPROVED KETO INGREDIENTS

HEALTHY FATS

Almond butter, unsweetened

Almond flour

Almond milk, unsweetened

Almond oil

Avocado

Avocado oil

Beef tallow

Butter

Cheese (blue cheese, cheddar, cream cheese, Colby, feta, mozzarella, provolone, ricotta, Swiss, etc.)

Coconut, shredded and unsweetened

Coconut aminos

Coconut cream (full-fat)

Coconut milk, unsweetened

Coconut oil

Chocolate, dark (90 percent cacao or higher), sugar-free

Cream, heavy

Cream, sour

Ghee

Lard

Mayonnaise

Milk, unsweetened almond

Milk, unsweetened coconut

Nuts (almonds, Brazil nuts, cashews, hazelnuts, macadamia nuts, peanuts, pecans, pili nuts, pistachios, walnuts)

Oils (coconut, extra-virgin olive, macadamia nut, sesame, walnut)

Olives

Peanut butter, natural no-sugar-added

Seeds (pumpkin, sesame, sunflower)

PROTEINS

Bacon, uncured, nitrite-free, sugar-free

Beef, fatty cuts

Beef, ground

Beef jerky (no sugar added)

Beef ribs

Beef roast

Bratwurst

Broth (beef, chicken)

Chicken, dark cuts with skin on

Duck

Eggs

Egg white protein powder

Fish (bass, carp, flounder, halibut, mackerel, salmon, sardines, trout, tuna)

Goose

Ham

Hot dogs (uncured)

Kielbasa

Liverwurst

Pepperoni

Pheasant

Pork (chops, ribs, roast)

Pork rinds

Quail

Salami

Sausage

Shellfish (crab meat, mussels, oysters, scallops, shrimp)

Steak (fattier cuts are better, like rib eye)

Turkey

Veal

HEALTHY CARBOHYDRATES

Artichokes
Arugula
Asparagus
Berries (blackberries,
    blueberries, raspberries,
    strawberries)
Bok choy
Broccoli
Brussels sprouts
Cabbage
Cauliflower
Celery
Chicory greens

Cranberries
Cucumbers
Eggplant
Garlic
Green beans
Jicama
Kale
Leeks
Lemon
Lettuce
Lime
Mushrooms
Okra

Onions
Peppers
Pumpkin
Radishes
Rhubarb
Scallions
Shallots
Snow peas
Spinach
Squash, spaghetti
Tomatoes
Watercress
Zucchini

FLAVORINGS

Coconut aminos
Extracts (such as LorAnn
    Naturals flavoring oils)
Hot sauce (Frank's RedHot,
    Tabasco)
Soy sauce
Stevia
Vanilla
Vinegar (apple cider,
    balsamic, sherry)
Worcestershire sauce

SPICES, HERBS, AND BAKING INGREDIENTS

Allspice
Baking powder
Baking soda
Basil
Celery seed
Chili powder
Cilantro
Cinnamon
Coriander
Cumin
Curry paste
Curry powder
Dill

Garlic
Ginger
Marjoram
Mustard seed
Nutmeg
Oregano
Paprika
Parsley
Pepper (black, cayenne)
Salt (sea, Himalayan)
Tarragon
Thyme
Turmeric

KETO-FRIENDLY THICKENING AGENTS

Guar gum and xanthan gum are excellent thickening agents.

Flour Replacement Guide

Amount of guar gum to use per 1 cup gluten-free flour:

- Cookies—¼ teaspoon
- Cakes—¾ teaspoon
- Muffins: 1 teaspoon
- Breads: 1 teaspoon

Amount of xanthan gum to use per 1 cup gluten-free flour:

- Cookies—¼ teaspoon
- Cakes—½ teaspoon
- Muffins—¾ teaspoon
- Breads—¾ teaspoon

Amount of glucomannan to use per 1 cup gluten-free flour:

- Cookies—½ teaspoon
- Cakes—¾ teaspoon
- Muffins—1 teaspoon
- Breads—1 teaspoon

How to Thicken Liquids

Amount of guar gum to use per 1 quart liquid:

- Hot liquids (soups)—1 to 2 teaspoons
- Cold liquids (syrups)—1 to 2 teaspoons

Amount of xanthan gum to use per 1 quart liquid:

- Hot liquids (soups)—2 teaspoons
- Cold liquids (syrups)—2 teaspoons

Amount of glucomannan to use per 1 quart liquid:

- Hot liquids (soups)—2 teaspoons
- Cold liquids (syrups)—2 teaspoons

QUICK KETO SWAPS

INSTEAD OF	USE
all-purpose flour	nut flour (almond, coconut)
rice	cauliflower rice
potatoes	roasted radishes
pasta	veggie zoodles
taco shells	cheese shells or lettuce wraps
hamburger buns	lettuce wraps or Hamburger Buns (page 187)
bagels	Keto Bagels (page 196)
chips	Cheese Crackers (page 26), kale chips, zucchini chips, or pork rinds
lasagna noodles	thinly sliced zucchini
fruit	LorAnn Naturals flavoring oils to add flavor to anything you make!

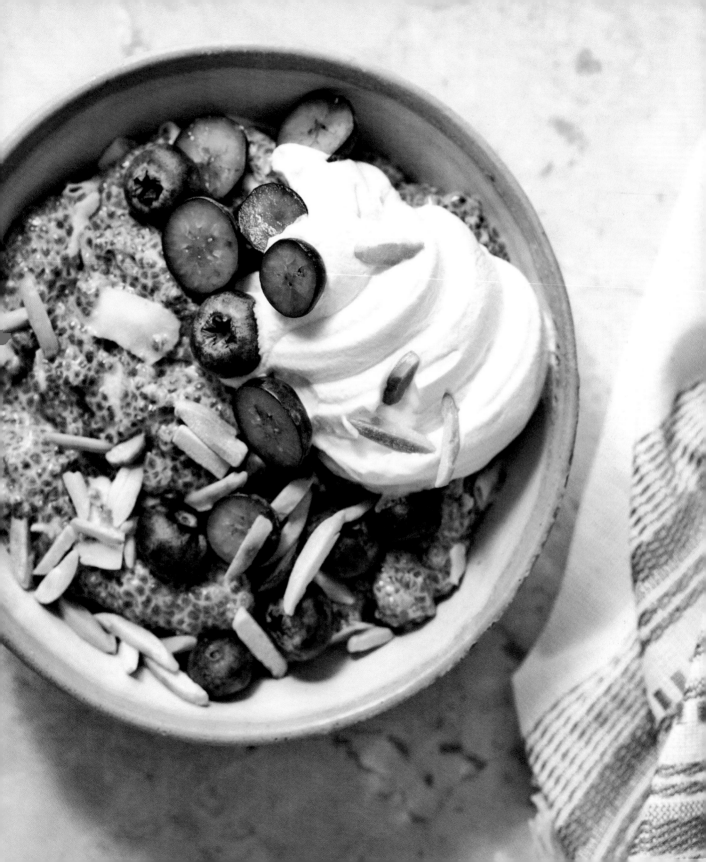

BEFORE YOU GET STARTED

Pantry Items

There are a few ingredients I recommend keeping in your pantry that will help you more easily adapt to the keto lifestyle.

SWEETENERS

There are several good sweeteners available that offer all the sweetness you want without the carbohydrates and calories. When you are at the store, pay attention to the labels. Many sweeteners look keto-friendly but they have extra processed ingredients that I don't recommend.

ERYTHRITOL: A natural sweetener found in pears, watermelon, and grapes. It is less sweet than sugar so it is often found mixed with other sweeteners like monkfruit.

Sukrin is a good brand that offers granulated, brown sugar, and confectioners' (aka icing sugar) varieties.

Swerve also offers granulated, brown sugar, and confectioners' varieties. It is a mix of erythritol and oligosaccharides. I love the taste of Swerve and use it all the time.

MONKFRUIT: This is a sweetener made from the juice of a small, round southeast Asian fruit.

My favorite brand is Lakanto, which can be found at many grocery chains. It comes in granulated ("Classic" on the Lakanto package), brown sugar ("Golden" on the Lakanto package), and powdered (aka confectioners') form and can be used 1:1 in place of sugar. There is a monkfruit extract in liquid form, but I don't use it in the recipes here.

STEVIA: Derived from the leaves of a plant native to Brazil and Paraguay, stevia also sweetens without calories. Pyure is my preferred brand and it offers both granulated and powdered (Bakeable Blend) varieties as well as liquid stevia.

ALTERNATIVE FLOURS

Flour with gluten is a no-no on the keto diet, but there are lots of other varieties to use instead.

COCONUT FLOUR: Made from dried coconut meat.

ALMOND FLOUR AND OTHER NUT FLOURS: Almost any nut can be made into flour, though almond flour is the most popular and the easiest to find at the store.

BONE BROTH

Made from the bones of beef or chicken, bone broth is cooked for at least 10 hours and up to 24 hours. It is high in collagen and has anti-inflammatory properties.

Kettle & Fire is my favorite brand. It really tastes great and it's a time-saver if you don't have time to make my Pressure Cooker Bone Broth (page 65).

BUTTER

This fat is used frequently on the keto diet, so it's good to buy the best you can afford.

Kerrygold has a higher butterfat content than other butters, plus it is free of growth hormones.

CHOCOLATE

It can be hard to find sugar-free chocolate that is naturally sweetened and free of artificial ingredients.

Lily's stevia-sweetened chocolate comes in a wide variety of bars, baking chocolate, and chocolate chips.

COLLAGEN

This is a protein made up of amino acids and can be purchased in powder form. It's also found in bone broth.

FIBER

Adding fiber to your diet helps maintain bowel health, lowers cholesterol, and controls blood sugar. It also aids in weight loss. Good sources of fiber include chia seeds, flaxseed, flax meal, and psyllium husk powder. You can also buy unflavored fiber in powder form and add it to beverages or recipes like Creamy Blueberry Ice Pops (page 215).

FLAVORINGS

If you want to add flavor without calories, a few drops of an oil flavoring can do the trick, but it's important that the flavoring you use includes only natural ingredients.

LorAnn Naturals is a wonderful brand with lots of flavors to choose from.

KETCHUP

Many bottled ketchups include sugar along with their other ingredients. I suggest making my Homemade Sugar-Free Ketchup (page 237).

AlternaSweets low-carb classic tomato ketchup is a good alternative ketchup if you can't make it yourself.

MAPLE SYRUP

You don't need to stop pouring syrup over your pancakes. My Homemade Maple Syrup (page 241) is sweetened with monkfruit.

ChocZero sugar-free maple syrup is sweetened with monkfruit and uses natural maple flavor.

MCT OIL

Short for medium chain triglycerides, MCT is a type of fat found in oils like coconut oil and some dairy products. This kind of fat is good because it goes from the gut to the liver where it is turned into ketones. You can buy the oil and add it to recipes to amp up the good fat in whatever you are eating.

PORK RINDS

These snacks are crunchy and delicious and a nice alternative to potato chips, which are not part of a keto diet. They are gluten-free, high protein, and free of carbs.

RO*TEL TOMATOES

This blend of tomatoes and chilies is delicious and adds lots of low-carb flavor. It comes in original, mild, and hot versions, which will appeal to pretty much any taste. They come in

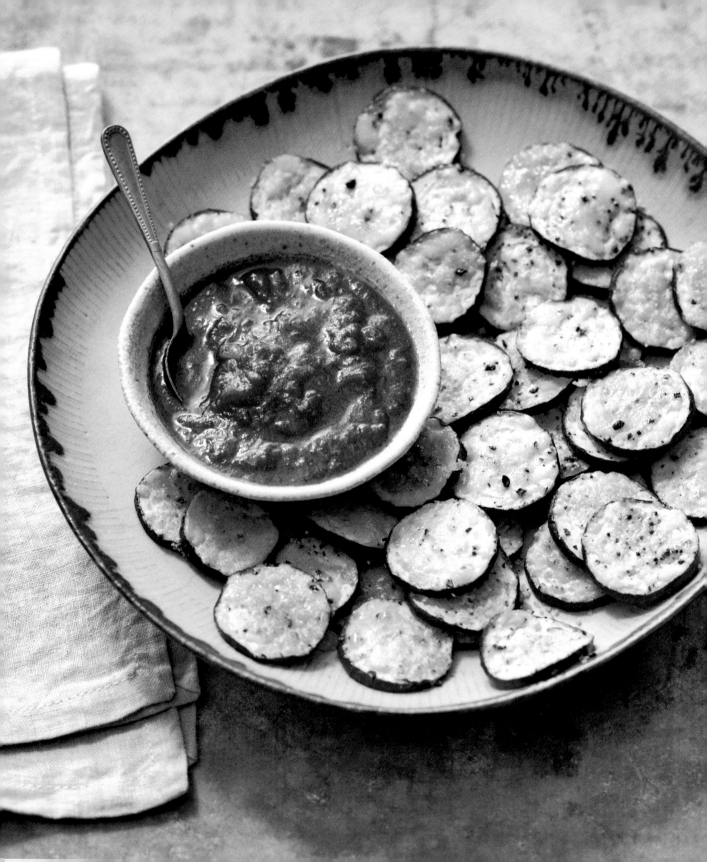

cans, so you can store them indefinitely in your pantry.

SALT
I use mostly table salt in the recipes but I also like pink Himalayan salt because, in addition to seasoning food, it has more than 84 minerals and trace elements that are good for you.

WHEY PROTEIN ISOLATE
A supplement that adds protein to your diet, whey isolates have a higher protein content than whey concentrate or whey hydrolysate, and they are almost completely dairy free and carbohydrate free.

XANTHAN GUM
This is a thickener and stabilizing agent that is often used to compensate for a lack of gluten in baked goods.

Kitchen Tools
The list below details kitchen gadgets, appliances, and equipment I use all the time. You don't need all of them to make the recipes, but they will make your life that much easier at mealtime.

AIR FRYER
An air fryer is a countertop appliance that works by circulating hot air around the food, much like a convection oven. The result is crisp "fried" chicken and other foods while using 70 percent less oil. I like to use it to make Buffalo Chicken Wings (page 108) and Parmesan-Crusted Pesto Pork Chops (page 127). These fryers are also speedy!

BAGEL/DONUT PAN
This pan helps form equally sized Keto Bagels (page 196).

BAKING SHEETS
You should have at least one and ideally two large baking sheets for making cookies and keto breads.

BLENDER
I use a blender all the time. My favorite is the Nutri Ninja Pro, which is small enough to fit on the countertop and powerful at 900 watts.

CAST-IRON SKILLET
This is my favorite pan because it goes from the stovetop to the oven and back again.

ELECTRIC PRESSURE COOKER OR INSTANT POT
I use the 6-quart Instant Pot Duo, which serves my family of four perfectly. If you've ever forgotten to defrost a meat for dinner, the pressure cooker is a lifesaver! My favorite thing to pressure cook is spaghetti squash.

FOOD PROCESSOR
Making cauliflower rice or nut flour is easy with this appliance.

MANDOLINE
This handy little tool is great for cutting vegetables very thinly. If you can't afford a spiralizer, this is the next best thing.

MILK FROTHER

A powerful handheld blender, the frother is battery operated and fantastic for blending a Fatty Coffee (page 39).

MINI MUFFIN PAN

Just the right size for making Fauxtato Tots (page 172).

SILICONE MATS

Nonstick mats that work like parchment but can be reused. They are especially good for rolling out dough without slipping around. After using, clean with warm water and a soft cloth.

SLOW COOKER

This is a great way to cook on a hot day without turning on the oven. Throw ingredients in the slow cooker in the morning and come home to a fully cooked dinner after work.

SPIRALIZER

This is an essential tool for making zoodles, aka zucchini noodles. I highly recommend you buy one. You can use a mandoline or a vegetable peeler, but a spiralizer is the fastest.

WHOOPIE PIE PAN

Although not essential, this makes it much easier to make keto breads, hamburger buns, or cheese chips uniform in size.

KETO IN REAL LIFE

Going to Restaurants While on the Keto Diet

I remember the struggle all too well in the beginning. I was overwhelmed with information and constantly trying to find hidden labels and ingredients in the foods I loved at my local restaurants. Over time, I've learned exactly what I can and can't have without much worry or stress. Let me tell you the easy way to eat at your favorite restaurant: Think meats and veggies. If you think about those two things, you can pretty much pick apart any menu to find something that fits your ketogenic lifestyle.

There is one problem that I still face today. It can be difficult to find restaurants that use real butter or healthy oils. I've been half tempted to carry butter around with me if I didn't have a fear of it melting in my purse. It's only the more high-end restaurants that tend to have these ingredients on hand when requested.

So I've learned to stop worrying about the healthy fats when I'm eating out and just choose foods that are naturally higher in fat. For example, I will order a rib eye steak. There is lots of fat in a rib eye! I will also order dark meat instead of a chicken breast. Most of the time you can request a side order of steamed vegetables.

If you frequent fast food places, there are some healthier choices there too. Almost every fast food chain sells burgers. Most are even offering a low-carb solution by wrapping burgers in lettuce. If your fast food place specializes in chicken, order the grilled chicken. If they don't offer steamed veggies, just order the chicken on a bed of lettuce. I went to a cheesesteak place in the mall once and ordered a naked Philly cheesesteak on a bed of lettuce. It was delicious! A woman in line behind me saw what I ordered and got the same thing.

I don't frequent fast food restaurants very much anymore. When you become fat adapted, you can stretch your eating windows for longer periods of time. This will allow you to even skip meals sometimes without the hunger pains you were used to before doing the keto diet.

To this day, I think going to the movies is still a struggle. We've all been trained to eat while we watch movies. I've become very aware of that and to be honest, that's not the problem. The thing that gets me is the delicious smell of popcorn as you walk through the lobby. I've started eating before I go to the movies so I won't be as tempted and so far, it's working.

Traveling While on the Keto Diet

Traveling while doing the keto diet has its challenges too. While running through the airport there's no shortage of carbs and sugar in every shop and every restaurant. The good news is that more times than not, you can also find a coffee shop that has sugar-free options or a newsstand that has packages of peanuts, pickles, and sometimes even hard-boiled eggs. Most restaurants in the airport

serve either BBQ or burgers. Both of these options are great! Order the fatty cuts of meats (hello, moist brisket) with no BBQ sauce (they often contain added sugar), or a burger with cheese, tomatoes, and onions served on a bed of lettuce. If you are in an airport food court, you can get a bunless burger or a breakfast sandwich with sausage, egg, and cheese without the bread part. The options are definitely there! It won't be long before you are an expert at picking apart menus to find food that fits your busy lifestyle. It's well worth the effort!

Ditch the Scale

This subject is really important to me. It's been said over and over again to "trust the process" while doing the keto diet, and removing your scale helps you with that trust.

I have been tracking the ups and downs of my dieting attempts for years, and the stress of the scale is not worth it. Seriously.

I suggest you only weigh yourself once a month. That way you won't worry when the scale fluctuates in either direction during the process. Start by keeping a log of your weight and measurements, and only track these numbers on a monthly basis.

There are many reasons why your weight fluctuates for both men and women. I have found that no matter how hydrated I think I am or how well I've done on the diet plan, my weight will always go up a pound or two when I've been outside in the hot Texas sun enjoying a day or two at the lake. The scale always goes back to normal or lower after I return and temperatures are back to normal.

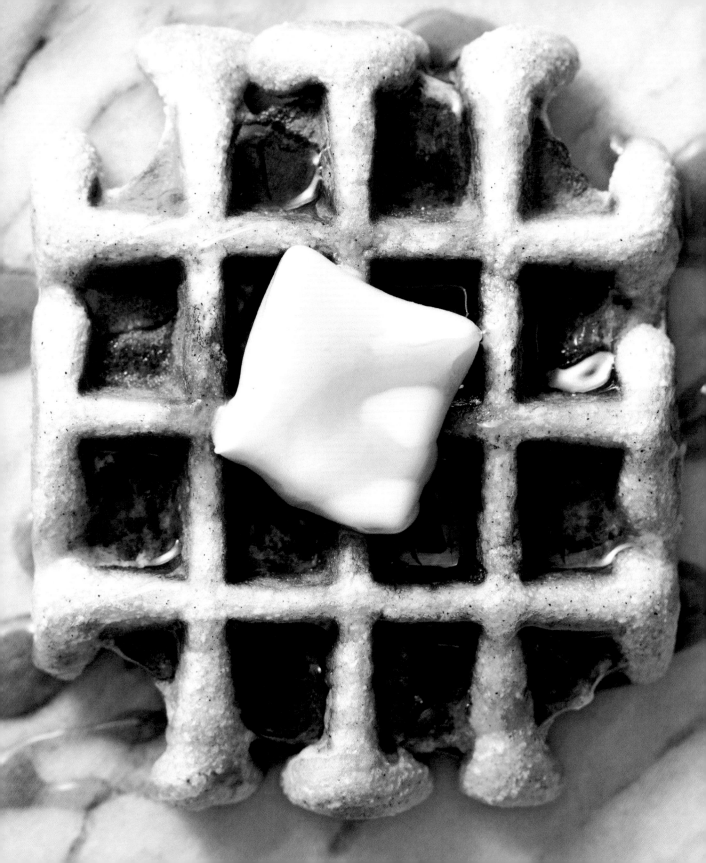

The other reason the scale may not move is that you might be constipated. Or for ladies, it could be that time of the month. If you track these numbers on a monthly basis instead of a daily basis you will see a trend in the right direction without the daily stress of going up or down a pound.

Keto in Social Situations

Social situations can be very difficult to maneuver when you are doing the keto diet. In the beginning, I would make sure I ate ahead of time before attending a party if I didn't know what was on the menu.

I would offer to bring a tray of food too. That way I could make sure there would be something keto-friendly at the party without putting the burden on the host and often without my non-keto friends even knowing. A meat and cheese tray—an "anti-pasta"—with tomatoes, cheese, artichoke hearts, and sliced meats is a perfect choice.

Intermittent Fasting

Maybe you've been eating a strict keto diet and you are either not losing weight or you've stopped losing weight? That was my situation for about 6 months, and I stopped counting after that because it was so frustrating to be eating the same foods that helped me lose 50 pounds but then to suddenly stop losing weight. This is where intermittent fasting really helped me.

I first heard about it from Dr. Jason Fung, author of *The Obesity Code,* and Dr. Annette Bosworth—they inspired me to look further

into it. Intermittent fasting is when you confine your eating to certain times of the day. Because your cortisol rises in the early morning hours, it's important to consume foods early and then avoid eating in the evening. This was really hard for me at first because, until then, I never ate breakfast, and sometimes I didn't eat lunch either.

To start intermittent fasting, the basic idea is to have a 12-hour period in which you don't eat. This will bring you into a state of autophagy, in which the body will start to consume its own tissue. In extreme cases like starvation, that would be very bad, but if your body is in that state intermittently, has nothing to digest, and gets no calorie intake, it will become very efficient. It will go through a process that looks at each cell in the body and either gets rid of it or makes it work at its most efficient. It's a sort-of "cleanup" process that readies the body for when you eat again in the morning. So even though I was still following the diet, I stopped losing weight because even on a low-calorie diet, the body tends to store calories and fat. But when you take in no calories, the body is forced into autophagy, when it uses what it already has instead of storing it, and that's when the body will start to lose weight again. I am not a doctor, so for a more detailed explanation, go to DietDoctor .com and see what Dr. Fung has to say about it, or go to bozmd.com for Dr. Boz's take on it.

When I began intermittent fasting, I didn't change the foods I was eating but, instead, I changed the time of the day those foods were consumed. That turned out to be the key to getting the scale moving again. Today, I stop eating anywhere from 4 to 6 p.m. every day, then I make sure I don't have my morning cup of coffee until 12 hours later. During the fast, I only drink water with some pink Himalayan salt if I feel hungry, which I was surprised to find really curbs my hunger! The other benefit of fasting for me is that I battle with insulin resistance, and a 12-hour fast every day allows my liver to use up all the glucose stored from the foods I consume. And by fasting in the evening hours, I'm supporting the speed in which my metabolism works, which is much more slowly than during the day. It turns out the biggest lesson I've learned by doing this is that success doesn't always come from what you eat, but when.

If you find yourself stuck in your weight loss journey like I did, try intermittent fasting. Losing additional weight is only a side benefit to all the health benefits this offers. You'll be able to control your blood sugar, boost your metabolism, fight inflammation, and improve your blood pressure, triglycerides, and cholesterol levels. You'll have more energy and just feel really good.

SAMPLE MEAL PLAN

I have put together a sample weekly meal plan that is very similar to how I eat each week so you can get an idea of how to plan what to eat each day. One thing I often do is double a recipe so that I'll have leftovers for the next day. It's not always easy to make dinner every night of the week. Sometimes, it really helps to have something in the refrigerator that only needs to be reheated in the microwave when you are too busy to cook. And with leftovers in the fridge, you're less likely to be tempted by processed convenience foods that are definitely not part of the keto diet.

I recommend that you plan your meals a week in advance and make sure you have the ingredients on hand, which will make following the diet that much easier.

	BREAKFAST	LUNCH	DINNER	SNACK/DESSERT
SUNDAY	Fatty Coffee (page 39), tea, or bone broth Creamy Keto Skillet Eggs (page 4)	Creamy Cucumber Salad (page 56)	Braised Beef Short Ribs (page 117) with Cauliflower-Creamed Spinach (page 168)	Low-Carb Chocolate Fudge (page 205)
MONDAY	Fatty Coffee, tea, or bone broth Bacon, egg, and cheese on a Low-Carb Biscuit (page 184)	Cheeseburger Salad (page 59)	Easy Oven-Baked Pork Ribs (page 131)	Lazy Keto Chips (page 33) with Guacamole (page 34)
TUESDAY	Fatty Coffee, tea, or bone broth French Toast Bake (page 11)	Thai Coconut Pumpkin Soup (page 71) with Cheese Crackers (page 26)	Mongolian Beef and Broccoli (page 119)	Sugar-Free Candied Pecans (page 35)
WEDNESDAY	Fatty Coffee, tea, or bone broth Quick One-Minute Muffin (page 13)	Leftover Mongolian Beef and Broccoli	Cheeseburger Salad	
THURSDAY	Fatty Coffee, tea, or bone broth Quick Blender Chocolate Protein Shake (page 21)	Parmesan Zucchini Crisps (page 176)	Garlic-Butter Rib Eye Steak Strips (page 114) with a small side salad and ranch dressing	Raspberry-Lemon Cupcakes (page 216)
FRIDAY	Fatty Coffee, tea, or bone broth Breakfast Granola Crunch (page 18)	Keto Bagel (page 196) with cream cheese	Garlic-Cilantro Grilled Chicken (page 105) with Prosciutto-Wrapped Cabbage (page 166)	
SATURDAY	Fatty Coffee, tea or bone broth Keto Pancakes (page 9)	Simple Chicken Salad with Balsamic Dressing (page 58)	Keto Italian Soup (page 76) with Cheese Crackers	Cosmopolitan (page 51)

1
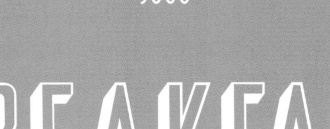
BREAKFAST

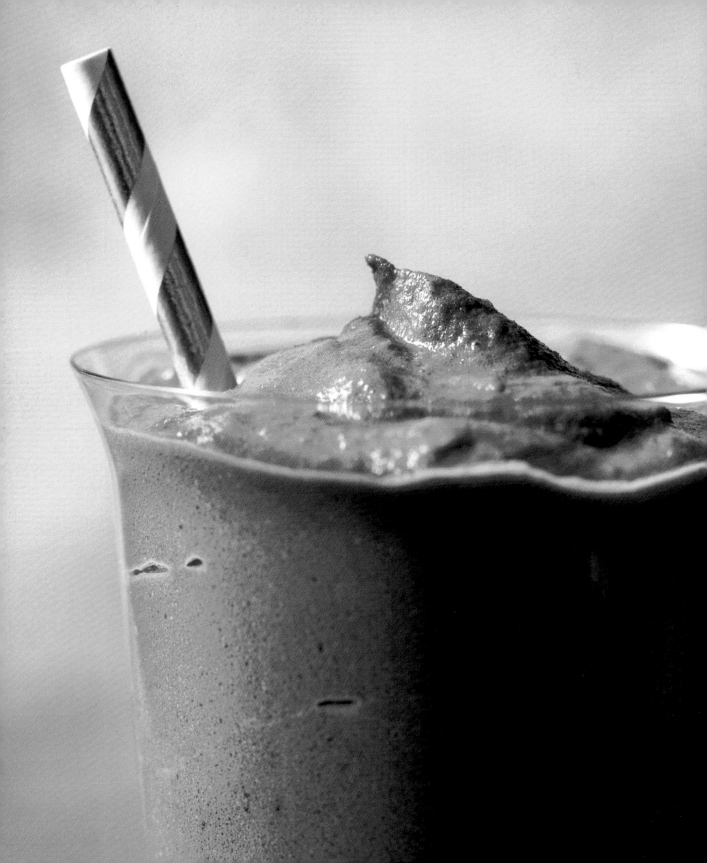

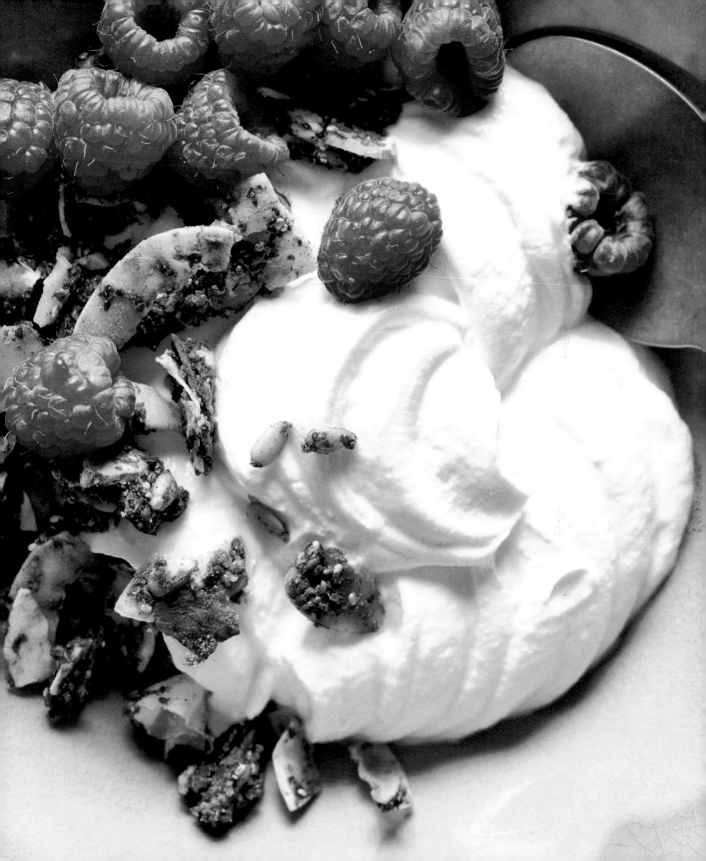

Cream gives these eggs the fat balance you need while keeping carbs low. And they make the creamiest, most delicious eggs ever, so much more interesting than everyday scrambled eggs. I love making them in my cast-iron skillet because it goes so easily from stovetop to oven.

CREAMY KETO SKILLET EGGS

MAKES 4 SERVINGS

PREHEAT the oven to 375°F.

POUR the olive oil into a 10-inch cast-iron skillet. Add the cream, salt, and pepper and bring to a simmer over low to medium heat, stirring constantly. Turn off the heat and stir in the parsley and dill. The mixture will start to thicken at this point. Crack each egg directly into the hot cream mixture.

TRANSFER the skillet to the oven and bake for about 8 minutes, until the yolks are cooked to your desired consistency. Sprinkle the bacon over the top and serve.

MAKES 4 SERVINGS

- 2 tablespoons extra-virgin olive oil
- ½ cup heavy cream
- ½ teaspoon salt
- ¼ teaspoon black pepper
- 2 tablespoons chopped fresh parsley
- 1 tablespoon chopped fresh dill
- 8 to 10 large eggs
- 4 slices sugar-free nitrite-free bacon, cooked and crumbled

NUTRITIONAL INFO (PER SERVING)
CALORIES 349, **FAT** 29.8 g, **PROTEIN** 17.3 g, **CARBS** 3.5 g, **FIBER** 0.4 g

VARIATION
Instead of crumbled bacon, try crumbled sausage, chorizo, or diced ham. I also love minced fresh chives sprinkled over the top.

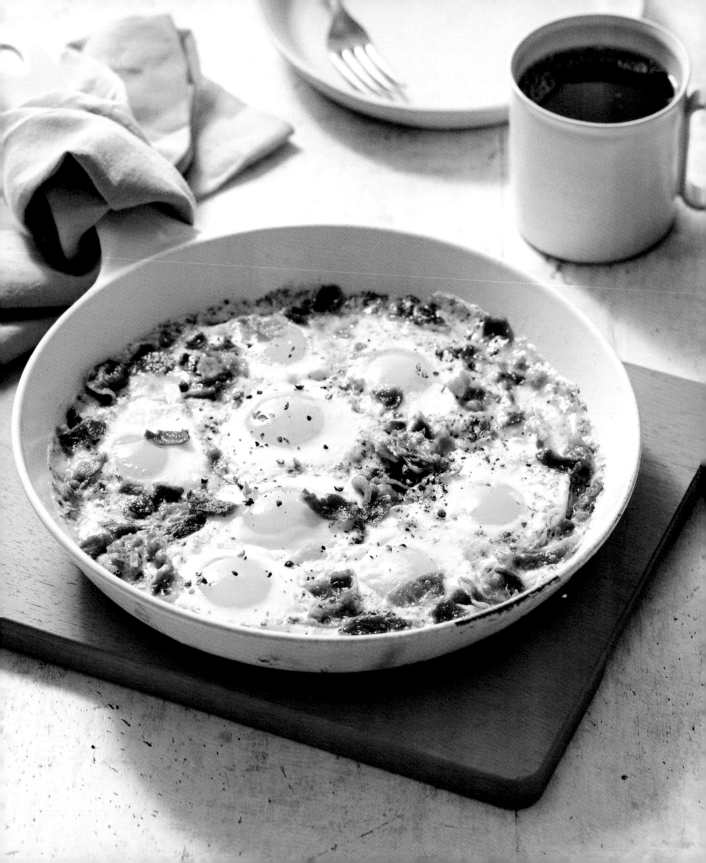

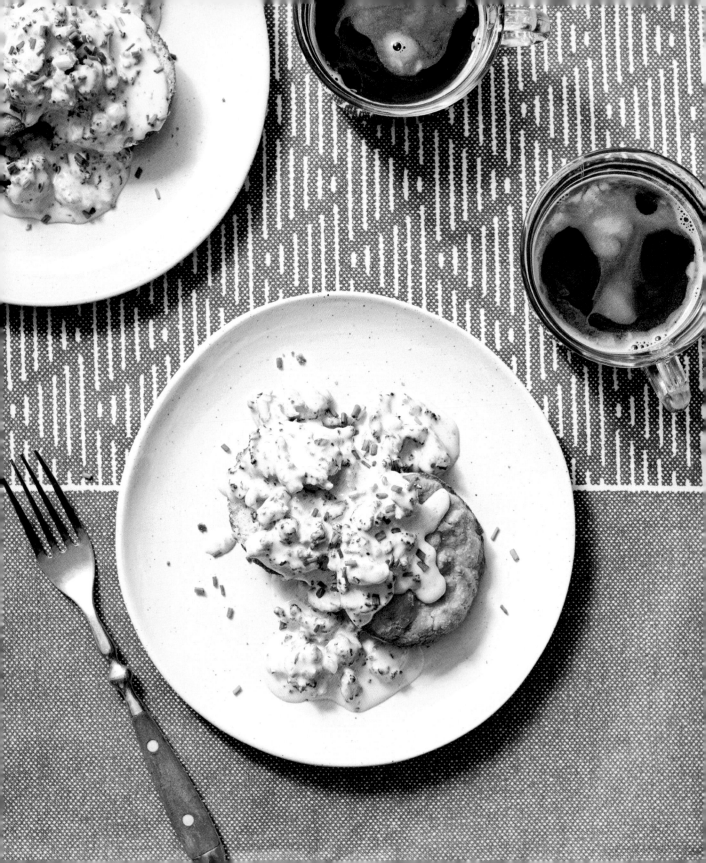

Serve with scrambled eggs on the side and you'll have a hearty keto-friendly breakfast that will keep you full for a long time.

BISCUITS WITH SAUSAGE GRAVY

IN a large skillet, cook the sausage meat over medium heat, breaking it up with a wooden spoon, until browned. Don't drain the fat. Add the cream cheese and stir until the mixture is combined and the cream cheese is melted. Stir in the cream and bring to a simmer. Add 2 tablespoons water and the xanthan gum, stir to combine, and continue to cook until the mixture forms a thick gravy, 1 to 2 minutes. Taste the sausage gravy and season with salt and pepper if needed.

CUT each biscuit in half and place on plates. Top with the sausage gravy and chopped chives, if using, and serve.

NUTRITIONAL INFO (PER SERVING)
CALORIES 537, **FAT** 47.8 g, **PROTEIN** 21.5 g, **CARBS** 8.7 g, **FIBER** 2.7 g

MAKES 8 SERVINGS

~~~~

1 pound bulk pork sausage

3 ounces cream cheese

1 cup heavy cream

1 teaspoon xanthan gum

Salt

Black pepper

8 Low-Carb Biscuits
   (page 184)

OPTIONAL TOPPING

chopped chives

VARIATION
For an extra layer of flavor, add ¼ cup chopped onion and a minced clove of garlic to the sausage before adding the cream cheese. You can also add a fried egg to each biscuit and then top with the sausage gravy.

This savory casserole is perfect for serving large groups; you can even double it if needed and simply bake it in two pans. Try it the next time you host a brunch. If you prefer a less spicy casserole, substitute 1 chopped green bell pepper for the jalapeños.

SPICY SAUSAGE AND EGG BREAKFAST CASSEROLE

PREHEAT the oven to 350°F. Spray a 9- by 13-inch baking pan with cooking spray.

IN a large skillet over medium-high heat, cook the sausage, breaking it up with a wooden spoon, until browned, about 8 minutes. Drain any excess grease. Add the cream cheese and cream, mix together, and cook for another 5 minutes, until the mixture is creamy. Remove from the heat.

IN a medium bowl, mix together the eggs, jalapeño, onion powder, parsley, and pepper. Spoon the sausage mixture into the egg mixture and mix together. Pour the mixture into the prepared baking pan. Sprinkle the cheese over the top, if using.

BAKE for 25 to 30 minutes, until the top is golden brown and the center is thoroughly cooked.

NUTRITIONAL INFO (PER SERVING)
CALORIES 403, **FAT** 31.9 g, **PROTEIN** 24.2 g, **CARBS** 4.2 g, **FIBER** 1 g

MAKES 6 SERVINGS

1 pound bulk pork sausage

4 ounces cream cheese

¼ cup heavy cream

6 large eggs

2 jalapeno peppers (fresh or pickled), diced

1 teaspoon onion powder

1 teaspoon chopped fresh parsley

½ teaspoon black pepper

½ cup shredded Colby or cheddar cheese, optional

If you are just starting out on the keto diet, know that you can still make foods you love—like these pancakes—and not feel like you are missing out on anything. Amp up the good fats by serving with a side of bacon.

KETO PANCAKES

MAKES 5 PANCAKES (5 SERVINGS)

PREHEAT a griddle.

COMBINE the cream cheese, eggs, coconut flour, vanilla, cinnamon, and salt in a blender and blend on high until smooth, about 1 minute. Alternatively, you can beat the ingredients in a bowl with an electric mixer until smooth, about 3 minutes.

MELT the butter on the griddle and spread it around with a spatula. Pour spoonfuls of batter onto the griddle and cook until bubbles form and start to pop. Flip and continue to cook until browned.

IF you like, serve with maple syrup or blueberry sauce.

2 ounces cream cheese

2 large eggs

2 tablespoons coconut flour

1 teaspoon vanilla extract

$\frac{1}{8}$ teaspoon ground cinnamon

$\frac{1}{8}$ teaspoon salt

1 tablespoon butter

OPTIONAL TOPPINGS

Homemade Maple Syrup (page 241) or other sugar-free maple syrup, Blueberry Sauce (page 243)

NUTRITIONAL INFO (PER SERVING)
CALORIES 172, **FAT** 14 g, **PROTEIN** 6.4 g, **CARBS** 4.6 g, **FIBER** 1.8 g

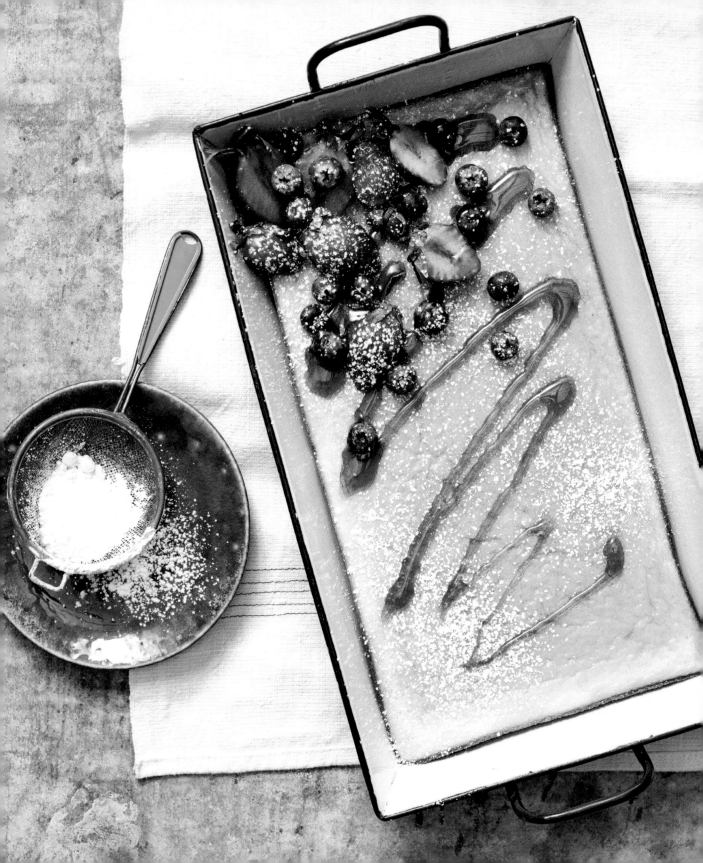

This recipe tastes just like real French toast—but without all the guilt! Drizzle your favorite sugar-free syrup over the top and you are in for a real treat. See below for ideas on changing up the flavor, and the Variations for fresh fruit ideas and an ingenious French Toast Roll.

FRENCH TOAST BAKE

PREHEAT the oven to 350°F. Spray a 7- by 11-inch baking pan with cooking spray.

COMBINE the eggs, butter, cream cheese, sweetener, and cinnamon in a blender and blend on high for about 1 minute, until smooth. Alternatively, you can beat the ingredients in a bowl with an electric mixer for about 3 minutes.

POUR the mixture into the prepared baking pan and bake for 40 minutes, until it's golden brown on the top. Cut into 4 pieces and serve.

PLACE any leftovers in a zip-top plastic bag and store in the refrigerator for up to 5 days. Reheat in the microwave.

NUTRITIONAL INFO (PER SERVING)
CALORIES 364, **FAT** 34.7 g, **PROTEIN** 16.3 g, **CARBS** 3 g, **FIBER** 0.1 g

MAKES 6 SERVINGS

~~~~

8 large eggs

8 tablespoons butter

8 ounces cream cheese

½ cup monkfruit powdered sweetener

¼ teaspoon ground cinnamon

OPTIONAL TOPPING

powdered stevia or Swerve confectioners' sweetener

FLAVORING OILS

LorAnn Naturals flavoring oils are a great way to add flavor (but not calories) to French toast and other savory and sweet dishes. Instead of the cinnamon, add 5 drops of one of the flavoring oils listed below. I particularly like the lemon and banana cream flavors.

- Vanilla
- Cinnamon
- Blueberry
- Strawberry
- Coconut
- Cheesecake
- Banana Cream
- Apple
- Lemon

(continued)

(French Toast Bake continued)

VARIATIONS

BLUEBERRY BREAKFAST BAKE: Omit the cinnamon and sprinkle 1 cup blueberries on top of the mixture before baking.

BLUEBERRY LEMON BREAKFAST BAKE: Omit the cinnamon and add 1 teaspoon lemon juice and 1 teaspoon grated lemon zest to the egg mixture. Sprinkle 1 cup blueberries on top of the mixture before baking.

RASPBERRY BREAKFAST BAKE: Omit the cinnamon and sprinkle 1 cup raspberries on top of the mixture before baking.

RASPBERRY LEMON BREAKFAST BAKE: Omit the cinnamon and add 1 teaspoon lemon juice and 1 teaspoon grated lemon zest to the egg mixture. Sprinkle 1 cup raspberries on top of the mixture before baking it.

FRENCH TOAST ROLLS: Divide the mixture among the cups of a 6-cup muffin tin and bake for 20 minutes at 350°F until the center is completely done.

This is an excellent recipe to make in a time crunch! Serve with a pat of butter and spread a little sugar-free jelly on it for a satisfyingly sweet treat. Ground sunflower meal can be found in your local health food store and online.

QUICK ONE-MINUTE MUFFIN

SPRAY a microwave-safe cup or mug with cooking spray.

IN a small bowl, combine the egg, sunflower meal, cream, Truvia, vanilla, and salt and mix well. Pour into the prepared cup and heat in the microwave oven for 1 minute. Top with the butter and eat right out of the cup.

NUTRITIONAL INFO (PER SERVING)
CALORIES 162, **FAT** 14 g, **PROTEIN** 6.7 g, **CARBS** 1 g, **FIBER** 0 g

VARIATION
Substitute ground flaxseed meal for the sunflower meal. Add another tablespoon cream to adjust for the flaxseed, which is a bit drier than sunflower meal.

MAKES 1 SERVING

1 large egg

¼ cup ground sunflower seed meal

1 tablespoon heavy cream

1 packet (¾ teaspoon) Truvia

½ teaspoon vanilla extract

1 pinch salt

1 teaspoon butter

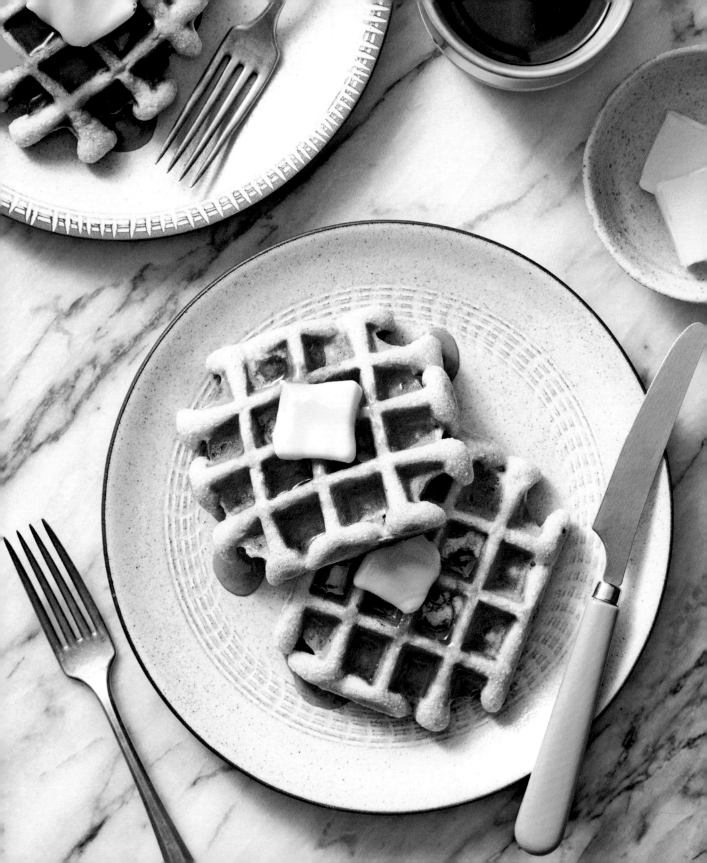

These are very filling so don't be surprised if you can only eat half of one. Save the rest for tomorrow or share with a friend. Instead of maple syrup, you can top with Blueberry Sauce (page 243), or serve with sliced strawberries.

FLUFFY KETO WAFFLES

**MAKES 4 WAFFLES
(4 SERVINGS)**

~~~

PREHEAT a waffle iron according to the manufacturer's instructions. Spray the waffle iron with cooking spray.

COMBINE the cream cheese, eggs, melted butter, coconut flour, stevia, baking powder, vanilla, and cinnamon, if using, in a blender and blend on high until smooth, about 1 minute. Alternatively, you can beat the ingredients in a bowl with an electric mixer until smooth, about 3 minutes.

POUR about ¼ cup of the batter onto the hot waffle iron. The batter will spread only a little bit, unlike conventional waffle batter, so spread it out a little with a spoon before closing the lid. Cook until browned. Repeat to make 4 waffles.

TOP with butter and maple syrup and enjoy.

4 ounces cream cheese

4 large eggs

1 tablespoon butter, melted

¼ cup coconut flour

1 tablespoon powdered stevia

1½ teaspoons baking powder

1 teaspoon vanilla extract

¼ teaspoon ground cinnamon, optional

Butter for serving

Homemade Maple Syrup (page 241) or other sugar-free syrup

NUTRITIONAL INFO (PER SERVING)
CALORIES 229, **FAT** 18.2 g, **PROTEIN** 9.6 g, **CARBS** 6.6 g, **FIBER** 2.9 g

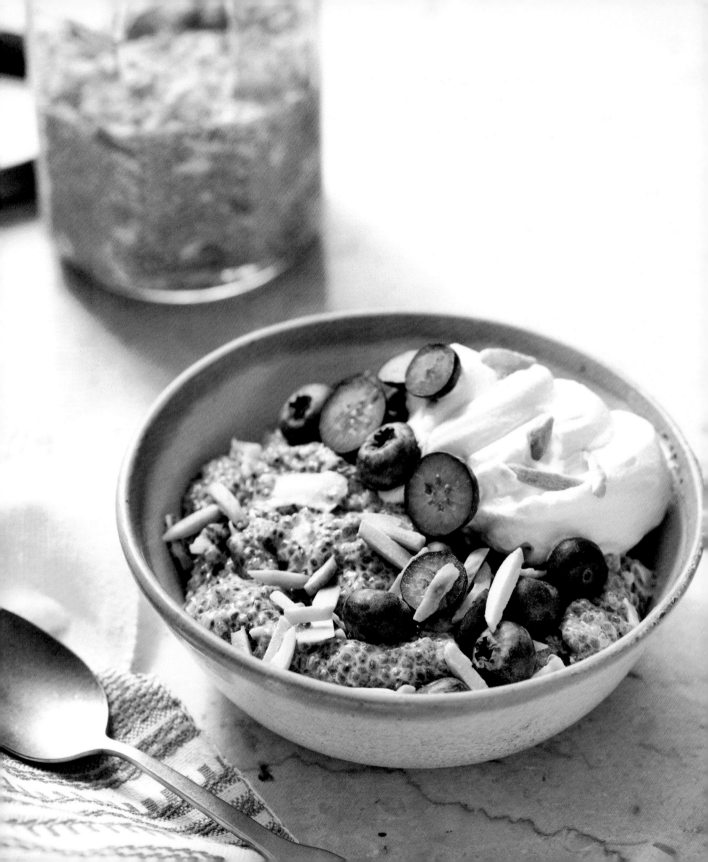

I like to eat this cold, but you can also heat it in the microwave if you'd rather start the day with a warm cereal. It's very filling, so it's a great choice if you have a busy day planned. I like to make and store this in a large Mason jar because you can seal it with the lid and shake it up instead of mixing with a spoon.

OVERNIGHT FAUX OATMEAL

MIX all the ingredients together in a large bowl or large Mason jar with a lid. Cover and refrigerate for at least 6 hours or overnight.

IN the morning, mix it again and spoon into two bowls. Add the toppings of your choice and serve.

NUTRITIONAL INFO (PER SERVING)
CALORIES 260, **FAT** 19.5 g, **PROTEIN** 6.2 g, **CARBS** 19 g, **FIBER** 10.6 g

MAKES 2 SERVINGS

~~~

1 cup almond milk

½ cup coconut milk

½ cup chia seeds

¼ cup unsweetened shredded coconut

2 tablespoons powdered stevia or erythritol

¼ teaspoon vanilla extract

⅛ teaspoon pumpkin spice seasoning

⅛ teaspoon ground cinnamon

OPTIONAL TOPPINGS

fresh blueberries, slivered almonds, whipped cream

This granola serves as a keto breakfast when it's served in a bowl with almond or coconut milk. You can also serve it with whipped cream and raspberries. But I usually package it in small containers so I'll always have snacks ready to go.

BREAKFAST GRANOLA CRUNCH

PREHEAT the oven to 350°F. Line a baking sheet with parchment paper or a silicone mat.

IN a large bowl, combine the pecans, almonds, sunflower seeds, flaxseed meal, coconut flakes, maple syrup, and chia seeds and mix well. Spread the mixture on the prepared baking sheet and sprinkle with the cinnamon.

BAKE for 10 minutes, until golden brown. Let cool for 10 minutes. The granola will harden and become crunchy after it cools.

GRANOLA can be stored in a covered container at room temperature for up to 7 days. It can also be frozen, wrapped tightly in plastic wrap, for up to 4 months.

NUTRITIONAL INFO (PER SERVING)
CALORIES 252, **FAT** 21 g, **PROTEIN** 7 g, **CARBS** 7.9 g, **FIBER** 6.5 g

MAKES 6 (½-CUP) SERVINGS

~~~

½ cup pecans

½ cup almonds

½ cup sunflower seeds

5 tablespoons ground flaxseed meal

5 tablespoons coconut flakes

¼ cup Homemade Maple Syrup (page 241) or other sugar-free maple syrup

1 tablespoon chia seeds

½ teaspoon ground cinnamon

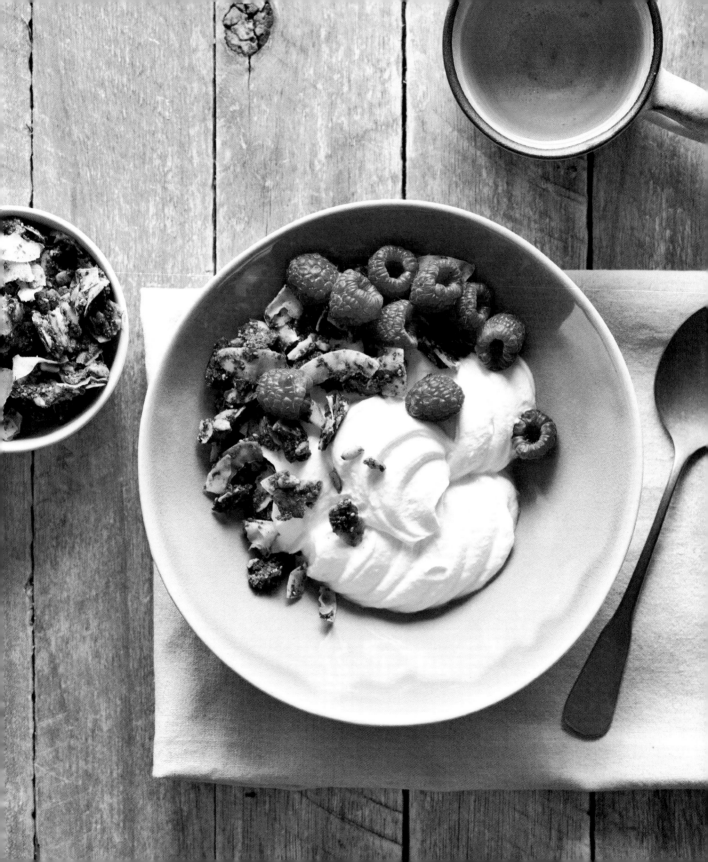

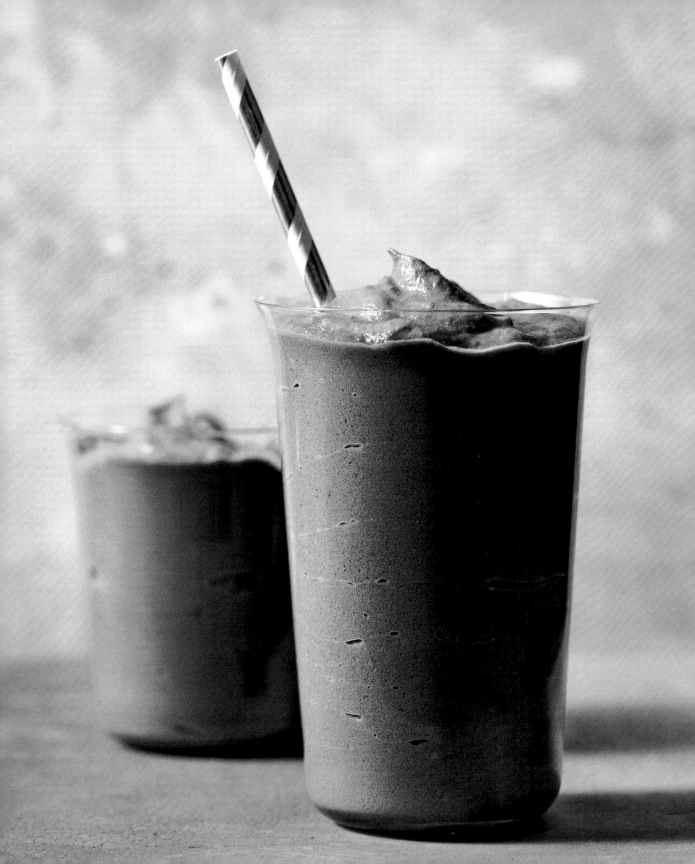

My kids love chocolate milk, so when I give them this for breakfast they are thrilled. Quest makes an amazing chocolate protein powder with no added sugars.

QUICK BLENDER CHOCOLATE PROTEIN SHAKE

COMBINE all the ingredients in a blender and blend on high until completely smooth, about 1 minute. Pour into a tall glass and serve.

NUTRITIONAL INFO (PER SERVING)
CALORIES 218, **FAT** 11.7 g, **PROTEIN** 18.5 g, **CARBS** 10.2 g, **FIBER** 2.9 g

MAKES 1 SERVING

~~~

- 2 cups unsweetened almond milk
- ½ cup ice cubes
- 3 tablespoons chocolate protein powder
- 1 teaspoon unsweetened cocoa powder

2

SNACKS, DRINKS & COCKTAILS

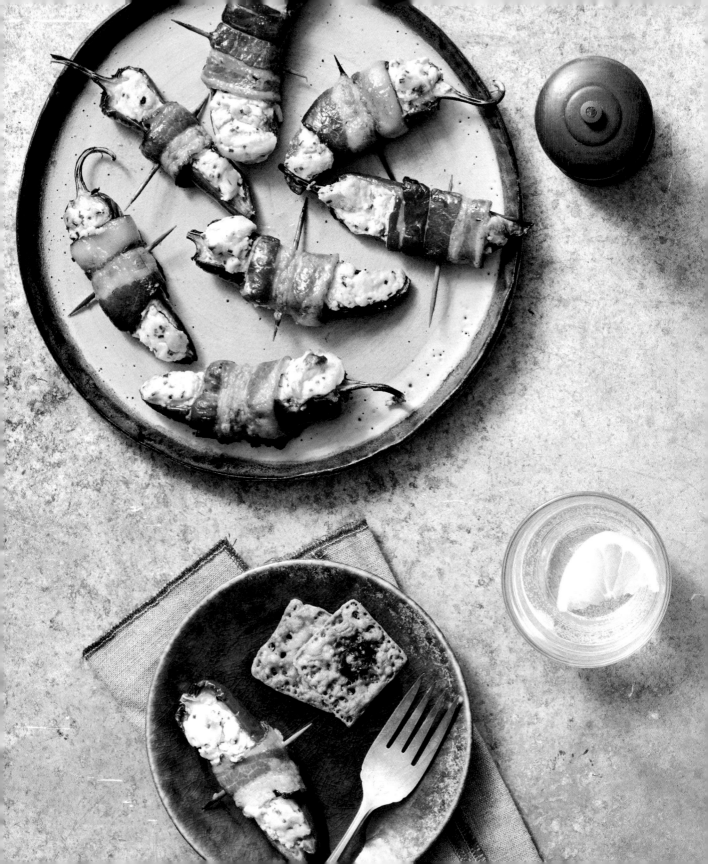

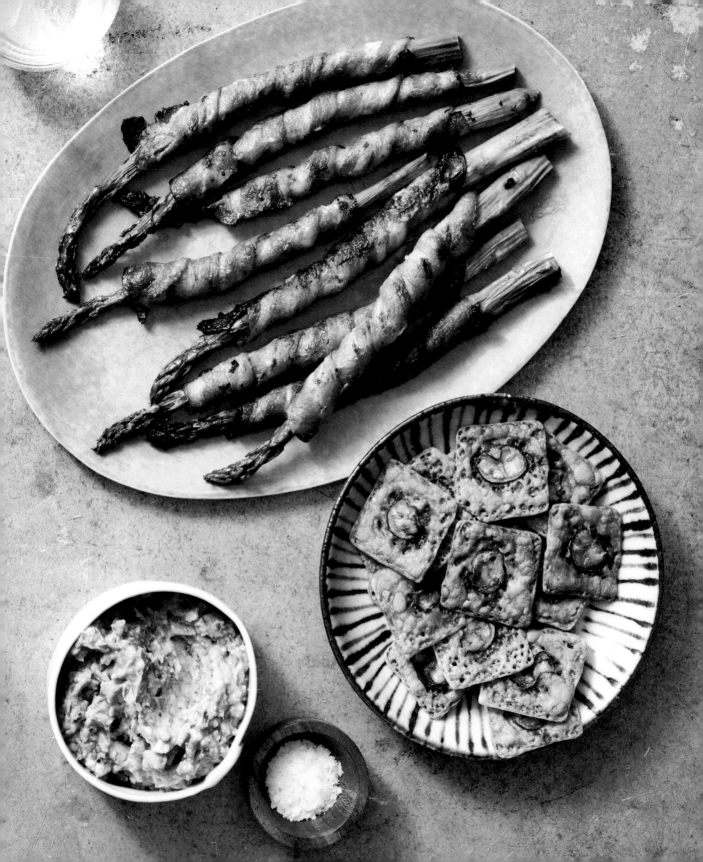

Put these out at parties or big game days and everyone will be very happy. This recipe works with almost any hard cheese: Swiss or cheddar is particularly good.

CHEESE CRACKERS

PREHEAT the oven to 450°F. Line a baking sheet with parchment paper or a silicone mat. Have a sheet of parchment paper ready.

MIX the grated cheese, cream cheese, and almond flour together in a microwave-safe bowl. Heat in the microwave oven for 1 minute. Stir until the mixture forms a dough. Alternatively, you can combine the ingredients in a saucepan and cook over medium heat just until the cheese melts and you can stir the mixture into a dough. Let cool for 5 to 10 minutes so when you add the egg, it won't start to cook.

ADD the egg, rosemary, and salt to the cheese mixture and combine until fully incorporated. If the cheese isn't melted enough or the dough is hard to mix, microwave for another 20 seconds and mix again.

PLACE the ball of dough on the prepared baking sheet and cover with the sheet of parchment paper. Using a rolling pin, roll out the dough until it's about ¼ inch thick. The thinner the dough, the crispier the crackers. The dough spreads easily so you can also press it out with your hands. Set aside the top sheet of parchment paper.

USING a pizza cutter, pastry wheel, or a sharp knife, cut the dough into 1-inch squares.

BAKE for 5 minutes, remove from the oven, cover with the sheet of parchment paper, and carefully flip over the dough. Continue to bake for another 5 to 6 minutes, until the crackers are crispy. Thicker dough may need to bake for 7 to 9 minutes. These can burn quickly so watch carefully.

LET the crackers cool for at least 5 minutes and serve.

MAKES 6 SERVINGS

∿∿∿

2 cups grated Parmesan-Romano cheese blend

2 ounces cream cheese

1 cup blanched almond flour

1 large egg

1 teaspoon chopped fresh rosemary

½ teaspoon salt

NUTRITIONAL INFO (PER SERVING)
CALORIES 263, **FAT** 20.7 g, **PROTEIN** 15.7 g, **CARBS** 5.6 g, **FIBER** 2.1 g

VARIATIONS
Try changing up the herb: Substitute 1 teaspoon dried basil, chives, garlic, dill weed, thyme, oregano, or a mix of several for the rosemary.

Chili powder gives the crackers a little kick. Use only ½ teaspoon unless you like things extra spicy.

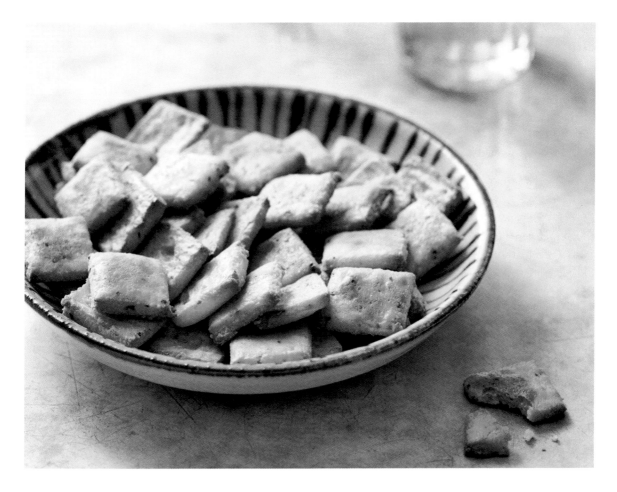

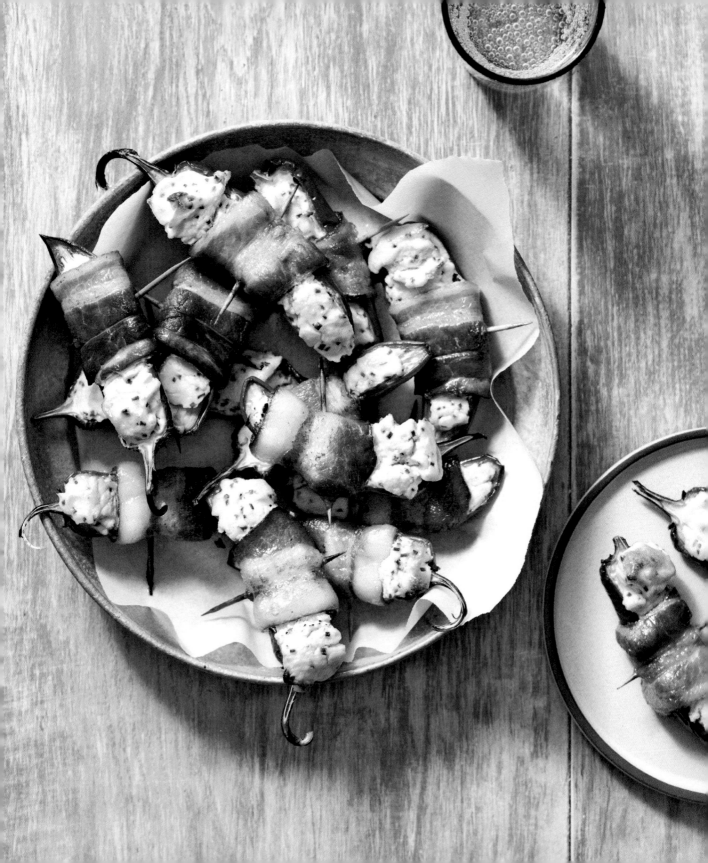

Almost every bacon you'll find at the grocery store has added sugar, so be sure to read the label closely. My favorite brand is Applegate Naturals. It's not only sugar-free, but nitrite-free as well. Poppers make a yummy snack but I've been known to eat these for lunch too. For the cream cheese, try one of the flavored versions. I like chive-onion.

JALAPEÑO–CREAM CHEESE POPPERS

MAKES 12 TO 16 SERVINGS

∿∿∿

6 to 8 fresh jalapeño peppers

8 ounces cream cheese

6 to 8 slices thick-cut sugar-free nitrite-free bacon, each cut in half to make 12 to 16 pieces

12 to 16 toothpicks, soaked in water for 15 minutes

PREHEAT the oven to 375°F. Line a baking sheet with parchment paper or a silicone mat.

CUT the jalapeños in half lengthwise and use a spoon to remove the seeds. Spoon about 1 tablespoon cream cheese into each half. Wrap with 1 piece of bacon. Use toothpicks to hold them together.

PLACE the poppers on the prepared baking sheet and bake for 25 to 30 minutes, until the jalapeño is tender and the bacon is crisp.

NUTRITIONAL INFO (PER SERVING)
CALORIES 93, **FAT** 7.5 g, **PROTEIN** 2.7 g, **CARBS** 4.3 g, **FIBER** 1.3 g

VARIATION
Mix ½ cup shredded cheddar, pepper Jack, or Colby cheese, or a mixture of them, with the cream cheese before stuffing the jalapeños to up the good fat—and the flavor!

You can easily adjust the spiciness factor by including the seeds from the jalapeño if you like your bread with a nice kick. If not, just leave them out. Pickled jalapeños are a good option too—they add more flavor with very little heat.

QUICK KETO JALAPEÑO CHEESE BREAD

PREHEAT the oven to 375°F. Line a baking sheet with parchment paper or a silicone mat.

COMBINE the mozzarella, Parmesan, and eggs in a bowl and mix until fully combined. Spoon the mixture onto the prepared baking sheet in 4 portions. Top each with slices of jalapeño.

BAKE for 15 to 20 minutes, until the cheese has fully melted and the bread begins to brown.

LET cool for 5 minutes and serve.

NUTRITIONAL INFO (PER SERVING)
CALORIES 156, **FAT** 9.5 g, **PROTEIN** 12.4 g, **CARBS** 5.2 g, **FIBER** 1.3 g

MAKES 4 SERVINGS

~~~~~

- 1 cup shredded part-skim low-moisture mozzarella cheese
- ½ cup grated Parmesan cheese
- 2 large eggs
- 2 fresh jalapeño peppers, seeded and sliced

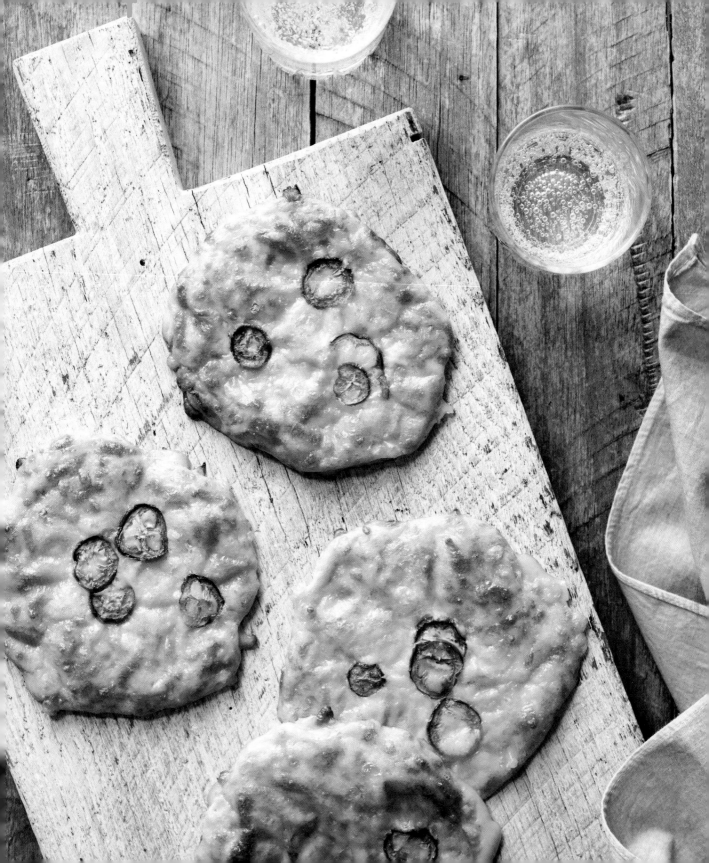

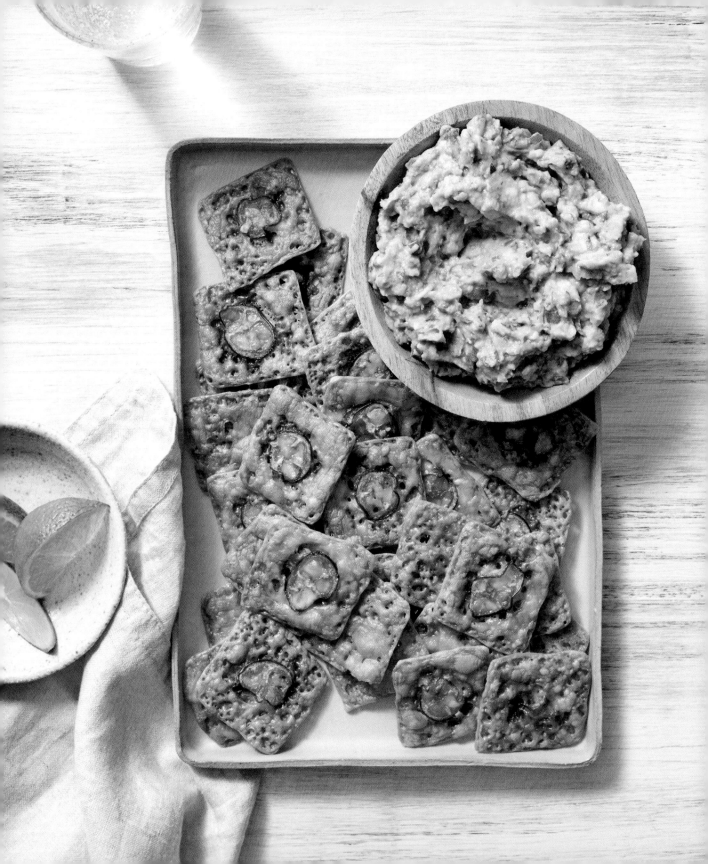

This recipe makes the best quick chips! Cut sliced cheese from the deli into 4 pieces, top with hot sauce, and bake. It couldn't get much easier, believe me. They are thick enough to dip into a bowl of Guacamole (page 34), or simply top them with a slice of jalapeño. Feel free to sprinkle one of the options from the Variations below over the cheese. Different cheeses create different chip flavors too. You will never get bored with this snack.

LAZY KETO CHIPS

MAKES 16 SERVINGS

PREHEAT the oven to 350°F. Line a baking sheet with parchment paper or a silicone mat.

ARRANGE the cheese slices on the prepared baking sheet, leaving a little space between each. Add a drop of Tabasco sauce on each slice and top with a slice of jalapeño, if using.

BAKE for about 15 minutes, until the cheese bubbles up. Let cool for at least 5 minutes. They will crisp up as they cool.

4 slices cheese (such as American, cheddar, or provolone), from the deli counter at the grocery store, cut into 1½-inch-square slices

Tabasco sauce, or other hot sauce

Jalapeño pepper slices (fresh or pickled), optional

NUTRITIONAL INFO (PER SERVING)
CALORIES 29, **FAT** 2.3 g, **PROTEIN** 1.6 g, **CARBS** 0.3 g, **FIBER** 0 g

VARIATIONS
Sprinkle 2 or 3 teaspoons sesame seeds, poppy seeds, pumpkin seeds, or sunflower seeds over the cheese slices and bake as directed.

Sprinkle 1 to 2 teaspoons oregano, herbes de Provence, or Italian seasoning over the cheese slices and bake as directed.

Jalapeño juice: That is the secret flavor weapon in my guacamole. You can get it from a jar of pickled jalapeños. A *molcajete* is a traditional Mexican stone mortar and pestle used to grind ingredients and often to make guacamole. If you don't have one, simply puree the jalapeño in a food processor instead. You can eat guacamole with your morning eggs, dollop it on salads, or serve with pretty much any protein you've chosen for your healthy fat. Serve with Lazy Keto Chips (page 33), pork rinds, or Cheese Crackers (page 26) for a perfect healthy snack.

GUACAMOLE

MAKES 6 SERVINGS

~~~

CRUSH the diced jalapeño, including the seeds, in a *molcajete* or a sturdy bowl with the back of a spoon until soft. Add the avocado, lime juice, tomato, onion, jalapeño juice, cilantro, salt, and garlic powder and mix with a spoon until evenly combined.

SERVE immediately.

1 fresh jalapeño pepper, diced with seeds

2 large or 3 small avocados, diced

Juice of ½ lime

3 tablespoons chopped tomato

3 tablespoons diced onion

2 tablespoons pickled jalapeño juice

2 tablespoons chopped fresh cilantro

½ teaspoon salt

¼ teaspoon garlic powder

NUTRITIONAL INFO (PER SERVING)
CALORIES 127, **FAT** 10.2 g, **PROTEIN** 2.5 g, **CARBS** 9.2 g, **FIBER** 5.9 g

It's always hard to stick to a diet around the holidays, so your friends and family will appreciate these candied pecans. They can indulge guilt-free.

SUGAR-FREE CANDIED PECANS

PREHEAT the oven to 325°F. Line a baking sheet with parchment paper or a silicone mat.

MELT the butter in a small microwave-safe bowl in the microwave oven. Add the erythritol, vanilla, and cinnamon and mix together.

PUT the pecans in a large zip-top plastic bag. Pour in the butter mixture, seal the bag, and shake gently until the pecans are completely covered with the butter mixture.

SPREAD out the pecans on the prepared baking sheet in one layer. Bake for 10 minutes, until the nuts are toasted and fragrant, checking frequently to make sure they don't burn. Let cool completely. The coating will harden as the pecans cool.

SERVE immediately, or put them in small decorative boxes for gifts.

MAKES 16 SERVINGS

~~~~

8 tablespoons butter

½ cup erythritol

1 teaspoon vanilla extract

1 teaspoon ground cinnamon

4 cups raw unsalted pecans

NUTRITIONAL INFO (PER SERVING)
CALORIES 198, **FAT** 20.7 g, **PROTEIN** 2.3 g, **CARBS** 3.7 g, **FIBER** 2.5 g

So versatile, these little treats make a nice party appetizer, or enjoy a few for a tasty lunch. The base is the Pocket Dough that I use in several recipes.

TACO BITES

PREHEAT the oven to 350°F. Have a silicone mat ready. Spray a 24-cup mini-cupcake pan with cooking spray (or use a nonstick pan).

IN a medium skillet, cook the ground beef over medium heat, breaking it up with a wooden spoon, until browned. Add the chili powder, cumin, salt, pepper, paprika, garlic powder, onion powder, oregano, and red pepper and stir to combine. Set aside to cool.

USING a rolling pin, roll out the dough to about ¼ inch thick on the silicone baking mat. Using a 3-inch round cookie cutter or a glass with the same diameter, cut out 24 rounds. Gather together the dough scraps, press together, reroll, and cut out more rounds if needed. Press one round into each well of the mini-cupcake pan. Spoon about 1 tablespoon of the seasoned ground beef into each dough-lined well. Top the ground beef with about 1 tablespoon shredded cheese.

BAKE for 10 to 15 minutes, until golden brown.

IF you like, serve with hot sauce, sour cream, and chopped green onions on the side.

MAKES 24 SERVINGS

~~~~~

1 pound ground beef

1 tablespoon chili powder

1½ teaspoons ground cumin

1 teaspoon salt

1 teaspoon black pepper

½ teaspoon paprika

¼ teaspoon garlic powder

¼ teaspoon onion powder

¼ teaspoon dried oregano

⅛ teaspoon crushed red pepper

Pocket Dough (page 143), omitting the garlic and onion powders

1½ cups shredded cheddar cheese

OPTIONAL TOPPINGS

hot sauce, sour cream, chopped green onions

NUTRITIONAL INFO (PER SERVING)
CALORIES 141, **FAT** 11.3 g, **PROTEIN** 7.5 g, **CARBS** 2.6 g, **FIBER** 0.9 g

---

VARIATION
Try different cheeses, like Monterey Jack, Colby, or provolone.

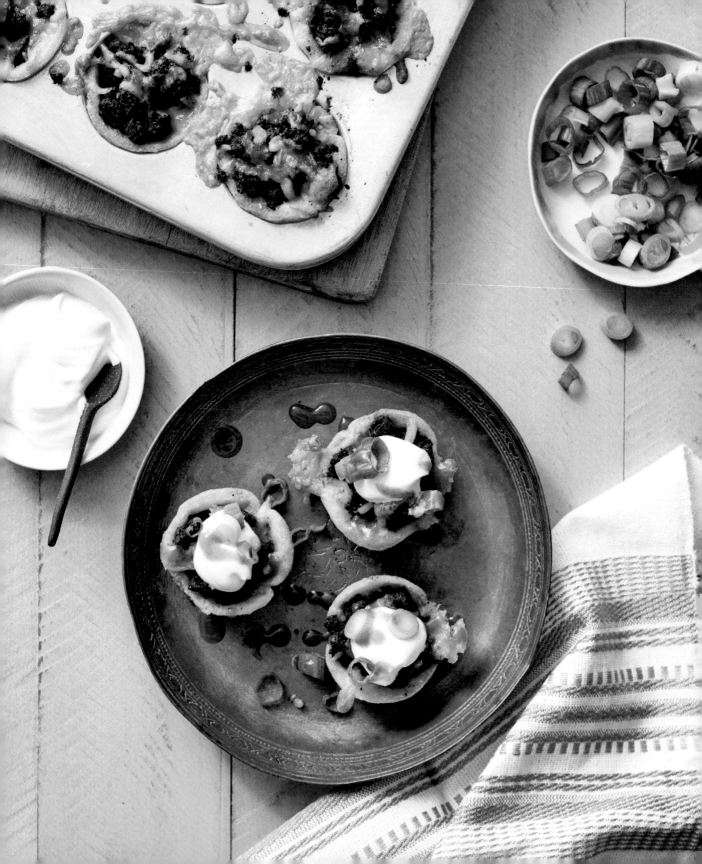

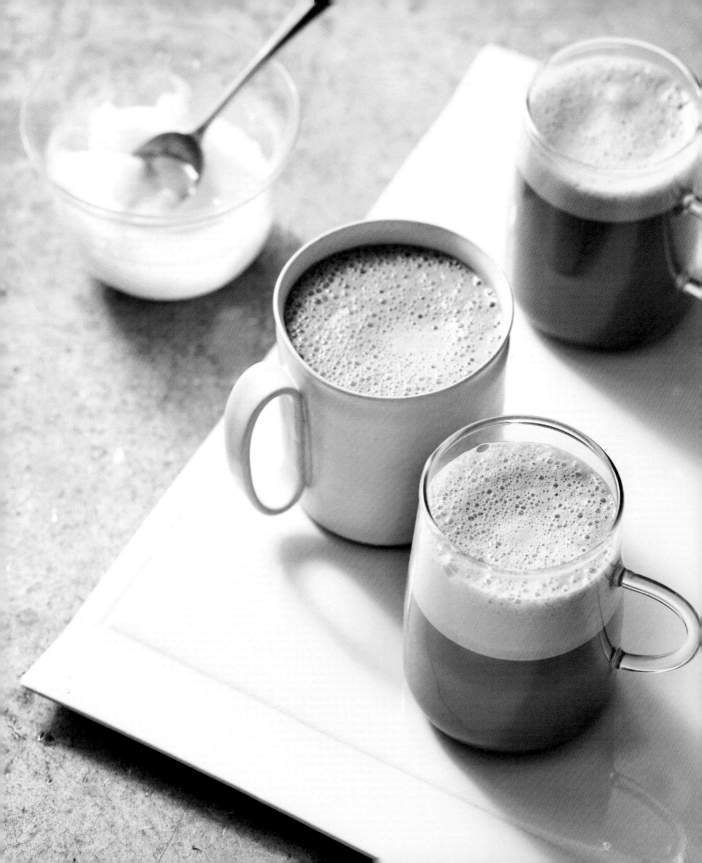

Most of the time I can skip breakfast completely when I enjoy a fatty coffee! The healthy fats—butter and MCT oil—in every cup keep me full and energized for hours. The trick to making this recipe smooth and frothy is to blend it in a high-speed blender to emulsify the fats and coffee into a rich and satisfying morning drink.

FATTY COFFEE

BLEND the coffee, coconut oil, butter, and stevia together in a blender on high for about 10 seconds. Make sure the lid is on tight—the coffee will be very hot. Remove the lid carefully, pour into a mug, and enjoy.

NUTRITIONAL INFO (PER SERVING)
CALORIES 225, **FAT** 25 g, **PROTEIN** 0.4 g, **CARBS** 0 g, **FIBER** 0 g

VARIATION
Add oil flavoring to this recipe to create different drinks. Peppermint is a favorite of mine around the holidays. A pinch of cinnamon is very nice too.

MAKES 1 SERVING

〜〜

- 8 ounces freshly brewed hot coffee, decaf or regular
- 1 tablespoon coconut oil or MCT oil
- 1 tablespoon butter
- 2 to 4 drops liquid stevia, optional

I created this recipe using nondairy milk, but you can use half-and-half or whole milk in its place. The butter gives the cocoa a luscious, rich mouthfeel that is out of this world.

BULLETPROOF HOT CHOCOLATE

IN a small saucepan over medium heat, whisk together the almond milk, cocoa powder, sweetener, and salt. Cook, stirring frequently, until the mixture just begins to boil. Lower the heat to low, add the butter, and mix together until the butter is melted. Pour into a mug and serve with a dollop of whipped cream.

NUTRITIONAL INFO (PER SERVING)
CALORIES 167, **FAT** 16.8 g, **PROTEIN** 2.4 g, **CARBS** 4.5 g, **FIBER** 1.6 g

MAKES 1 SERVING

~~~

- 8 ounces unsweetened almond milk or hazelnut milk
- 1 tablespoon unsweetened cocoa powder
- 1 tablespoon monkfruit sweetener
- Pinch of salt
- 1 tablespoon butter or coconut oil
- Whipped cream

I've used a mixture of cream and almond milk for the spiced latte, but you can use all whole milk or half-and-half—or go all nondairy and use the nut milk of your choice. Whatever you choose will taste great.

HOT CHAI LATTE

MAKES 1 SERVING

FOR THE CHAI SPICE

POUR 2 cups water into a medium saucepan set over high heat. Add the ginger, cloves, cardamom, cinnamon, star anise, vanilla, allspice, nutmeg, and sea salt and bring to a boil. Remove from the heat, add the tea bags, cover, and let steep for 45 minutes.

STRAIN the mixture through a fine mesh sieve and discard the solids. Let cool completely. Makes about 2 cups. The mixture can be stored in an airtight container in the refrigerator for up to 1 week.

FOR THE LATTE

COMBINE the cream, almond milk, and sweetener in a saucepan over medium-high heat, stirring frequently to dissolve the sweetener. When the mixture just starts to steam, but before it begins to boil, add ¼ cup of the chai spice, remove the pan from the heat, and stir to combine. Add more chai spice if you want a more pronounced spice flavor.

NUTRITIONAL INFO (PER SERVING)
CALORIES 316, **FAT** 32.9 g, **PROTEIN** 3 g, **CARBS** 5.4 g, **FIBER** 0 g

CHAI SPICE

1-inch piece peeled fresh ginger, cut into slices

5 whole cloves

5 cardamom pods

2 cinnamon sticks

2 whole star anise

1 teaspoon vanilla extract

½ teaspoon whole allspice

½ teaspoon freshly grated nutmeg

Pinch fine sea salt

3 black tea bags

LATTE

¾ cup heavy cream

½ cup almond milk

1 tablespoon monkfruit sweetener

VARIATION
Iced Chai Latte: Make the latte as instructed but let the milk mixture cool to room temperature before adding the chai spice. Fill a tall glass with ice, pour in ¼ cup chai spice, and mix together thoroughly.

Refreshing and tart, this is the perfect drink for a hot summer day.

STRAWBERRY LIMEADE

MAKES 6 SERVINGS

~~~

IN a microwave-safe bowl, stir together the sweetener and ½ cup water. Heat in the microwave oven in 30-second intervals, stirring each time, until the sweetener is dissolved, creating a simple syrup (see page 48).

IN a blender, puree the strawberries with 1 cup water, then press the mixture through a fine-mesh sieve, reserving the liquid and discarding the solids.

POUR the lime juice into a large pitcher. Add the simple syrup, pureed strawberries, and 4 to 5 cups cold water. Stir together, taste, and add more water or lime juice if needed.

SERVE in ice-filled glasses, garnished with a lime wheel or skewered strawberries.

½ cup monkfruit sweetener

2 cups fresh or thawed frozen strawberries

¾ cup fresh lime juice (from 8 or 9 limes)

Lime wheels or strawberries, for garnish

NUTRITIONAL INFO (PER SERVING)
CALORIES 23, **FAT** 0.2 g, **PROTEIN** 0.4 g, **CARBS** 6.6 g, **FIBER** 1.1 g

There are few drinks more refreshing than lemonade. Try mixing it with iced tea to create an Arnold Palmer.

LEMONADE

MAKES 8 SERVINGS

~~~

IN a microwave-safe bowl, stir together the sweetener and ¾ cup water. Heat in the microwave oven in 30-second intervals, stirring each time, until the sweetener is dissolved, creating a simple syrup (see page 48). Pour into a large pitcher.

ADD the lemon juice, 8 cups cold water, and the lemon slices. Stir together and serve in ice-filled glasses.

¾ cup monkfruit sweetener

1 cup fresh lemon juice
   (from 5 to 6 lemons)

Sliced lemons

NUTRITIONAL INFO (PER SERVING)
CALORIES 7, **FAT** 0.1 g, **PROTEIN** 0.1 g, **CARBS** 5.1 g, **FIBER** 0.1 g

VARIATION
To make an Arnold Palmer, mix together equal amounts Lemonade and brewed iced tea and stir to combine. You can experiment with the proportions to get the balance you like the best. Garnish with a lemon wheel.

AM I ALLOWED TO DRINK WINE OR A COCKTAIL ON THE KETO DIET?

The answer is yes! Just because you are living a keto lifestyle doesn't mean you can't have a glass of wine or a cocktail sometimes.

COCKTAILS: There are definitely types of alcohol that are better than others. When in doubt go for classic alcohols like vodka, whiskey, tequila, rum, and gin. Stay away from liqueurs, which are very high in sugar.

WINE: In general, the drier the better and go for white wine before red. For whites, try brut champagne and similarly styled sparkling wines, cava, and prosecco. If you don't want sparkling wine, look for Pinot blanc and Pinot grigio. Reds start out higher in carbs, with pinot noir coming in at about 3.4 grams per serving. Merlot, cabernet, and Syrah are just a little higher.

MIXERS: Be careful! Tonic is loaded with sugar. Instead, try mixing your drinks with sparkling water. And stay away from premixed cocktail helpers like margarita mix or Bloody Mary mix, which can blow your maximum carb allowance with one drink. Instead try my classic Margarita (page 48), which is made from scratch and comes in at 19 grams of carbs per cocktail, or my Keto Mary (page 50), with its crunchy bacon, olive, and cornichon garnish.

BEER: Most beer is generally pretty high in carbs, so it's best to avoid it.

Margarita, page 48 ▷

◁ Cosmopolitan, page 51

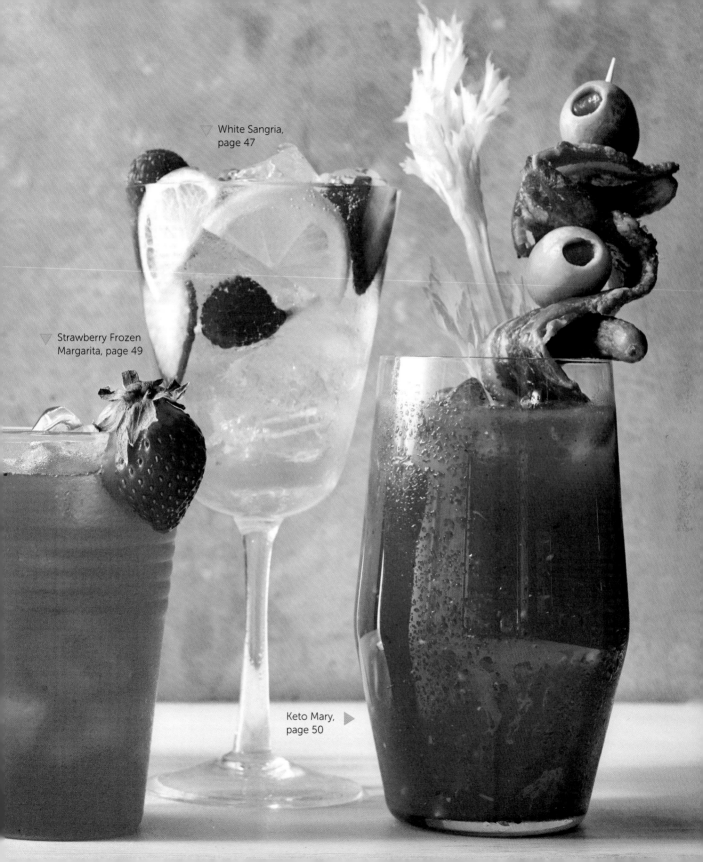

White Sangria, page 47

Strawberry Frozen Margarita, page 49

Keto Mary, page 50

Serve with Taco Bites (page 36) the next time you have a few people over.

RED SANGRIA

IN a large pitcher or punch bowl, stir together the wine, vodka, and sweetener until the sweetener is dissolved. Add the sparkling water and stir gently. Add the blueberries, blackberries, and raspberries and serve.

NUTRITIONAL INFO (PER SERVING)
CALORIES 194, **FAT** 1.1 g, **PROTEIN** 0.8 g, **CARBS** 17.2 g, **FIBER** 2.1 g

~~~

1 (750-milliliter) bottle dry red wine (such as Pinot noir)

8 ounces vodka

½ cup monkfruit sweetener

16 ounces sparkling water

1 cup fresh or frozen blueberries

1 cup fresh or frozen blackberries

1 cup fresh or frozen raspberries

The best way to enjoy this is with friends on a hot summer day.

WHITE SANGRIA

IN a large pitcher or punch bowl, stir together the wine, brandy, and sweetener until the sweetener is dissolved. Add the sparkling water and stir gently. Add the lemon and lime slices and the strawberries and raspberries and serve in ice-filled glasses.

NUTRITIONAL INFO (PER SERVING)
CALORIES 90, **FAT** 0.2 g, **PROTEIN** 0.4 g, **CARBS** 9.1 g, **FIBER** 1.4 g

〜〜〜

1 (750-milliliter) bottle dry white wine (such as pinot grigio)

8 ounces brandy

⅔ cup monkfruit sweetener

16 ounces sparkling water

2 lemons, sliced

2 limes, sliced

1 cup sliced strawberries

1 cup raspberries

Ice

A classic margarita usually has triple sec or Grand Marnier, which are not friendly with the keto diet. To get that orange flavor, I substitute a little orange-flavored sparkling water—the kind that adds just a little bit of flavor but no sugar or calories.

MARGARITA

MAKES 1 SERVING

~~~

Lime juice

Salt

Ice

2 tablespoons monkfruit sweetener

1½ ounces tequila

1 ounce lime juice

2 to 3 ounces sparkling water with orange essence

Lime wheel, for garnish

FOR the rim, pour the lime juice and salt in separate shallow bowls. Dip the rim of a rocks glass in the lime juice and then in the salt. Add ice to the glass and set aside.

IN a very small microwave-safe bowl, stir together the sweetener and 2 tablespoons water. Heat in the microwave oven for 15 seconds and stir until the sweetener is dissolved, creating a simple syrup. Microwave for 10 seconds longer if needed to dissolve the sweetener.

FILL a cocktail shaker with ice. Add the simple syrup, tequila, and lime juice and shake vigorously for several seconds. Pour into the rocks glass and top with sparkling water. Stir gently to combine. Garnish with a lime wheel and serve.

NOTE: *Monkfruit sweetener mixed with water makes an excellent simple syrup, but it's important to note that it tends to recrystallize when it cools, which is why I don't suggest making a big batch and storing it. It can be redissolved in a microwave in 15-second intervals and stirred to break up the crystals, if needed.*

NUTRITIONAL INFO (PER SERVING)
CALORIES 65, **FAT** 0.1 g, **PROTEIN** 0.6 g, **CARBS** 19.4 g, **FIBER** 0.2 g

VARIATIONS

MARGARITAS FOR EIGHT: Mix 1 cup monkfruit sweetener and 1 cup water together in a small bowl and microwave in 15-second intervals, stirring in between, until the sweetener is dissolved. In a large container with a tight-fitting lid, combine the simple syrup, 12 ounces tequila, and 8 ounces lime juice. Shake vigorously, pour into 8 ice-filled glasses, and top with soda water. Garnish with lime wheels.

STRAWBERRY FROZEN MARGARITA: Add the Margarita ingredients to a blender along with 5 to 6 strawberries and about 1 cup ice. Blend until slushy. Serve with skewered strawberries for garnish.

RASPBERRY FROZEN MARGARITA: Add the Margarita ingredients to a blender along with ½ cup raspberries and about 1 cup ice. Blend until slushy. Serve with skewered raspberries or a lime wheel.

I use a long wooden skewer to thread the bacon, olives, and cornichons for the garnish.

KETO MARY

MAKES 1 SERVING

∿∿∿

THREAD the cooked bacon onto a wooden skewer, alternating with olives and cornichons, the bacon weaving through like a ribbon. Set aside.

FILL a tall glass with ice and place the celery stalk in the glass.

IN a cocktail shaker with a lid, combine the tomato juice, vodka, Worcestershire sauce, sriracha, and horseradish, if using. Shake vigorously for several seconds and pour into the ice-filled glass. Top with a grind or two of salt and pepper. Place the bacon skewer into the drink and serve.

- 1 slice thick-cut sugar-free nitrite-free bacon, cooked
- Olives
- Cornichons
- Ice
- 1 stalk celery, trimmed with leaves intact
- 6 ounces unsweetened tomato juice
- 2 ounces vodka
- 1 teaspoon Worcestershire sauce
- 1 teaspoon sriracha
- 1 teaspoon prepared horse-radish, optional
- Pink Himalayan salt
- Black pepper

NUTRITIONAL INFO (PER SERVING)
CALORIES 236, **FAT** 3.6 g, **PROTEIN** 5.5 g, **CARBS** 14.1 g, **FIBER** 2.7 g

If Carrie Bradshaw had known about monkfruit sweetener, I like to think she would have made her cosmopolitan just like this one. Lightly sweet, not too tart, and pretty low in calories.

COSMOPOLITAN

IN a very small microwave-safe bowl, stir together the sweetener and 1 tablespoon water. Heat in the microwave oven for 15 seconds and stir until the sweetener is dissolved, creating a simple syrup (see page 48). Microwave for 10 seconds longer if needed to dissolve the sweetener.

IN an ice-filled cocktail glass, combine the simple syrup, vodka, and cranberry juice. Stir thoroughly and garnish with a lime wheel.

NUTRITIONAL INFO (PER SERVING)
CALORIES 129, **FAT** 0 g, **PROTEIN** 0 g, **CARBS** 4 g, **FIBER** 0 g

MAKES 1 SERVING

1 tablespoon monkfruit sweetener

Ice

2 ounces vodka

1½ ounces unsweetened cranberry juice

Lime wheel

Tonic is loaded with sugar, but if you cut the amount in half and replace it with sparkling water, you preserve the flavors without veering from your diet. This is a special treat.

GIN & TONIC

IN an ice-filled cocktail glass, combine the gin, tonic, and sparkling water and stir gently. Garnish with a lime wheel.

NUTRITIONAL INFO (PER SERVING)
CALORIES 21, **FAT** 0 g, **PROTEIN** 0 g, **CARBS** 5.4 g, **FIBER** 0 g

MAKES 1 SERVING

~~~

Ice

2 ounces gin

2 ounces tonic water

2 ounces sparkling water
 with lime essence

Lime wheel

It's not the holidays without eggnog, so here's a recipe that you can indulge in without falling off the keto wagon.

EGGNOG

MAKES 8 SERVINGS

~~~

4 large eggs, separated

½ cup monkfruit powdered sweetener

12 ounces heavy cream

8 ounces milk

1 teaspoon grated nutmeg, plus more for garnish

½ teaspoon ground cinnamon

1 teaspoon vanilla extract

8 ounces rum

Whipped cream, optional

IN a medium bowl, beat the egg yolks with an electric mixer until they lighten in color. Add the sweetener and continue to beat until thoroughly mixed. Set aside. Cover the egg whites and place in the refrigerator until ready to use.

IN a saucepan over medium-high heat, bring the cream, milk, nutmeg, and cinnamon to a boil. Remove from the heat.

WHILE whisking constantly, slowly add about ¼ cup of the hot milk mixture to the egg yolk mixture, then add the egg yolk mixture back into the hot milk and continue to whisk. Return the pan to the heat and cook until the mixture reaches 160°F. Remove from the heat, mix in the vanilla, and let cool to room temperature. Pour into a pitcher and refrigerate for at least 3 hours.

ABOUT 1 hour before serving, remove the egg whites from the refrigerator to warm to room temperature.

JUST before serving, whisk the rum into the chilled eggnog. Beat the egg whites with an electric mixer until they form stiff peaks. Add the whites to the eggnog and whisk until fully incorporated.

SERVE with a dollop of whipped cream, if using, and a grating of nutmeg.

NUTRITIONAL INFO (PER SERVING)
CALORIES 335, **FAT** 25.8 g, **PROTEIN** 6.1 g, **CARBS** 8.9 g, **FIBER** 0.8 g

3

SALAD
& SOUP

A spiralizer makes quick work of slicing the cucumbers into ribbons. This cool, refreshing salad is perfect for a backyard barbecue and pairs nicely with grilled chicken or ribs.

CREAMY CUCUMBER SALAD

IN a small bowl, mix together the sour cream, olive oil, vinegar, dill, sweetener, celery seed, salt, and pepper until the dressing is fully combined.

IN a serving bowl, toss together the cucumbers, radishes, and onion. Drizzle the dressing over the cucumber mixture and toss until well coated.

REFRIGERATE until ready to serve. This salad can get a little watery if it's left out at room temperature. If it does, drain the liquid and toss the mixture again.

NUTRITIONAL INFO (PER SERVING)
CALORIES 206, **FAT** 17.3 g, **PROTEIN** 3.8 g, **CARBS** 13.4 g, **FIBER** 3.9 g

MAKES 4 SERVINGS

~~~

¼ cup sour cream

¼ cup extra-virgin olive oil

2 tablespoons apple cider vinegar

¼ cup minced fresh dill

1 tablespoon Swerve confectioners' sweetener

1 teaspoon celery seed

1 teaspoon salt

½ teaspoon black pepper

2 cucumbers, peeled and thinly sliced

8 radishes, trimmed and sliced

½ cup diced onion

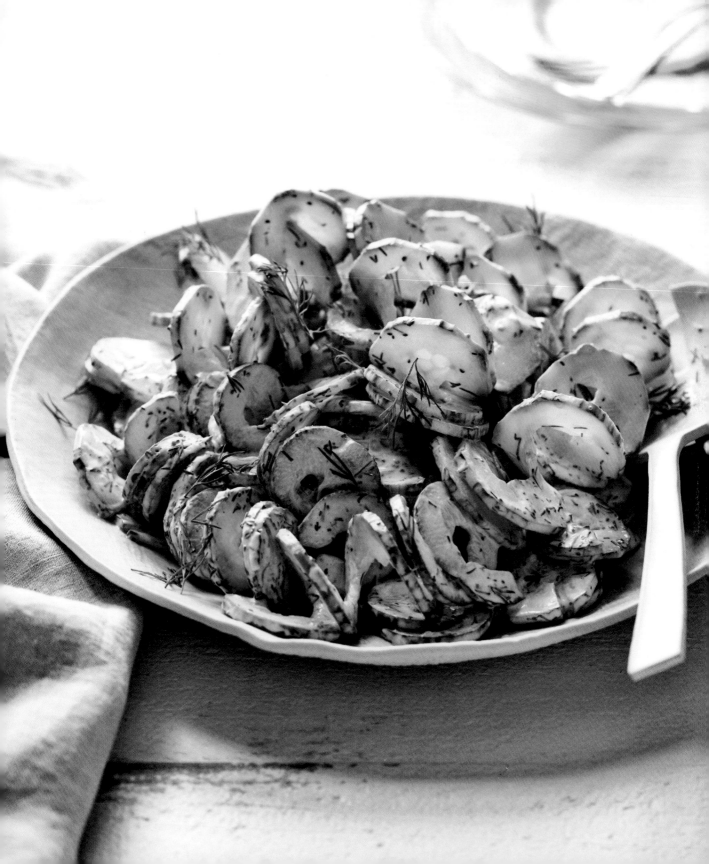

This hearty meal in itself doesn't require any sides. The balsamic dressing does double duty—it's a marinade for the chicken and a dressing to drizzle over the finished salad. You can use chicken breasts here, but chicken thighs have a higher fat count and are more tender, so use them if you can.

SIMPLE CHICKEN SALAD WITH BALSAMIC DRESSING

MAKES 4 SERVINGS

~~~

4 boneless chicken thighs, skin removed (reserve for frying, see Note)

¼ teaspoon salt

⅛ teaspoon black pepper

¾ cup Balsamic Dressing and Marinade (page 226)

4 slices sugar-free nitrite-free bacon

8 cups mixed salad greens

½ green bell pepper, diced

½ cup diced red tomato

½ cup diced onion

1 medium avocado, diced

¼ cup crumbled feta cheese

SEASON the chicken thighs with the salt and pepper. Place the chicken and ¼ cup of the dressing in a large zip-top plastic bag, seal, and marinate at room temperature for at least 20 minutes.

IN a skillet over medium heat, cook the bacon. Transfer to paper towels, leaving the bacon fat in the pan. Add the chicken thighs to the skillet and cook until they are no longer pink in the center, 5 to 7 minutes. Transfer the chicken to a cutting board, cut into slices, and set aside.

IN a large serving bowl, combine the salad greens, bell pepper, tomato, onion, and avocado. Top with the slices of chicken. Crumble the bacon and scatter over the chicken. Drizzle with the remaining ½ cup dressing and sprinkle with the feta.

A KETO TREAT: CRISPY CHICKEN SKIN

One of the most delicious keto snacks is crunchy, fried chicken skin. Lightly coat a skillet with oil and cook the skin from the chicken thighs over medium-high heat until golden and crispy. Let cool on a paper towel and sprinkle with salt before serving. These are so addictive you need no storage instructions.

NUTRITIONAL INFO (PER SERVING)
CALORIES 405, **FAT** 23.2 g, **PROTEIN** 36.8 g, **CARBS** 13.6 g, **FIBER** 6.1 g

A salad that is hearty enough to fill you up? Yes! Honestly, this one hardly feels as though it's low-carb at all.

CHEESEBURGER SALAD

MAKES 4 SERVINGS

IN a small bowl, whisk together 2 teaspoons water with the mayonnaise, sour cream, ketchup, relish, onion, vinegar, sweetener, hot sauce, and a pinch of salt. Set the dressing aside.

IN a medium skillet, heat the oil over medium-high heat. Add the onion and cook, stirring, until translucent, about 2 minutes. Add the ground beef and 1 teaspoon salt and cook, breaking the beef up with a wooden spoon, until browned, 6 to 7 minutes. Add the garlic and mix together. Remove the pan from the heat and set aside.

DIVIDE the romaine, tomatoes, and cheese equally among four large bowls or plates. Spoon the beef mixture equally over the salads. Drizzle each bowl with 2 heaping tablespoons dressing. Garnish with pickle slices, if using. Serve immediately.

NUTRITIONAL INFO (PER SERVING)
CALORIES 183, **FAT** 7 g, **PROTEIN** 19.8 g, **CARBS** 11.9 g, **FIBER** 3.4 g

2 tablespoons mayonnaise

2 tablespoons sour cream

2 tablespoons Homemade Sugar-Free Ketchup (page 237)

1 tablespoon pickle relish

1 tablespoon minced onion

1 teaspoon apple cider vinegar

1 teaspoon monkfruit sweetener

Dash hot sauce

Salt

2 teaspoons extra-virgin olive oil

1 large onion, chopped

1 pound ground beef

2 cloves garlic, minced

1 large head romaine lettuce, chopped

2 large ripe tomatoes, chopped

1 cup shredded sharp cheddar cheese

Dill pickle slices, optional

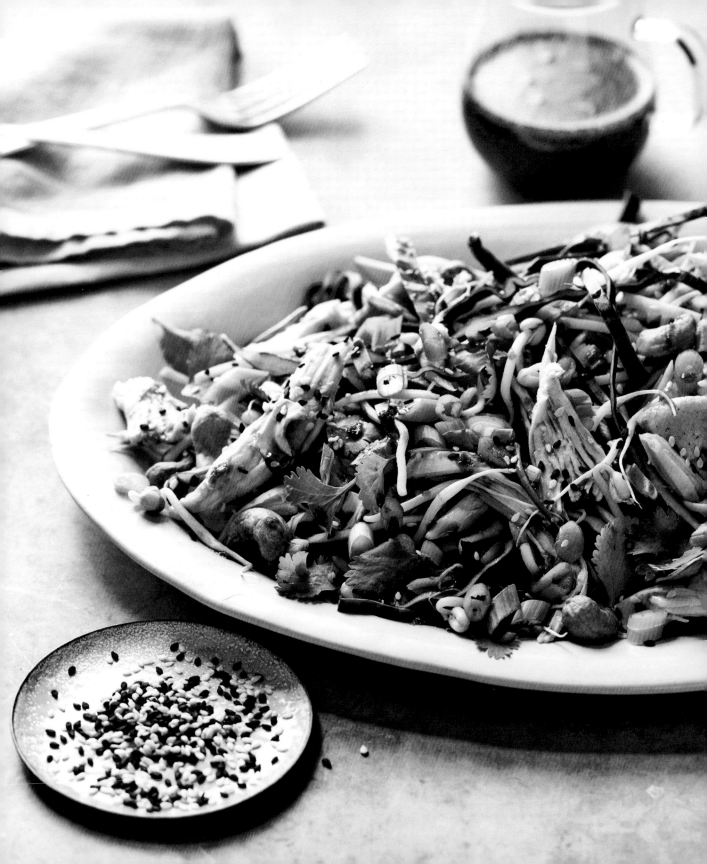

This recipe is an excellent quick dinner and a great way to use a cooked rotisserie chicken. You can also purchase precut shredded cabbage. Feel free to assemble the salad in the morning, then, just before serving, add the sesame dressing and toss to combine.

ORIENTAL CHICKEN SALAD WITH SESAME DRESSING

FOR THE SALAD

IN a large serving bowl, mix together the chicken, cabbage, broccoli, green onions, sprouts, cashews, and cilantro. Set aside.

FOR THE DRESSING

IN a bowl, whisk together the coconut aminos, sesame oil, vinegar, lime zest and juice, ginger, garlic, and chili sesame oil, if using.

JUST before serving, drizzle the dressing over the salad and toss to combine. Garnish with the sesame seeds.

NUTRITIONAL INFO (PER SERVING)
CALORIES 179, **FAT** 9.5 g, **PROTEIN** 17.1 g, **CARBS** 7.3 g, **FIBER** 2.4 g

MAKES 4 SERVINGS

CHICKEN SALAD
2 cups shredded cooked chicken
2 cups finely shredded red cabbage
1 cup shredded broccoli
½ cup thinly sliced green onions
½ cup bean sprouts
¼ cup cashews
¼ cup minced fresh cilantro

SESAME DRESSING
½ cup coconut aminos
1 tablespoon toasted sesame oil
1 tablespoon rice vinegar
1 teaspoon grated lime zest
1 tablespoon lime juice
½ teaspoon minced fresh ginger
½ teaspoon minced garlic
½ teaspoon chili sesame oil, optional
2 tablespoons sesame seeds

You can use metal or wooden skewers for grilling the shrimp. If using wooden skewers, soak them in water for about 20 minutes before using.

CHILI-LIME GRILLED SHRIMP SALAD

IN a medium bowl, mix together the lime zest, ¼ cup of the lime juice, the chili powder, paprika, and cumin. Add the shrimp, toss, and marinate at room temperature for 20 minutes.

PREHEAT a grill to medium heat.

THREAD the shrimp onto the skewers. Grill until the shrimp turns pink, 4 to 5 minutes per side. Remove the shrimp from the skewers and set aside in a bowl.

IN a separate bowl, make the dressing by combining the remaining ¼ cup lime juice, the olive oil, cilantro, salt, and pepper.

IN a large serving bowl, toss together the mixed greens, avocado, tomato, and onion. Top with the grilled shrimp and drizzle with the dressing.

NUTRITIONAL INFO (PER SERVING)
CALORIES 474, **FAT** 28.1 g, **PROTEIN** 48.3 g, **CARBS** 13 g, **FIBER** 6.4 g

MAKES 4 SERVINGS

∿∿∿

1 teaspoon grated lime zest

½ cup lime juice

1 tablespoon chili powder

½ teaspoon smoked paprika

½ teaspoon ground cumin

2 pounds medium shrimp, peeled and deveined

¼ cup extra-virgin olive oil

½ cup chopped fresh cilantro

½ teaspoon salt

¼ teaspoon black pepper

5 cups mixed salad greens

1 avocado, diced

½ cup diced tomato

¼ cup diced onion

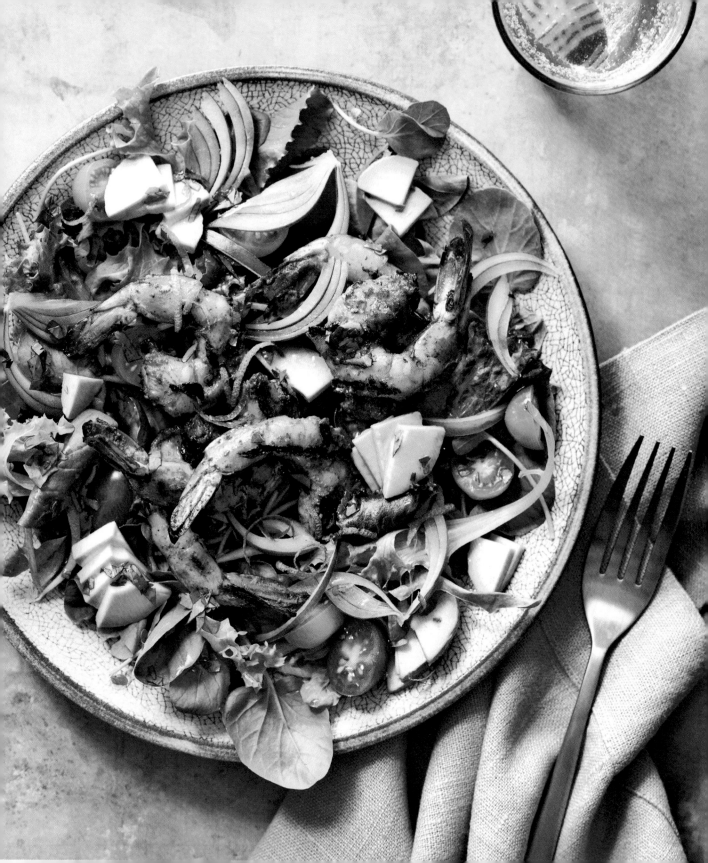

If you enjoy spicy foods, leave the seeds in the jalapeños. Avocado gives this tuna salad a wonderful creamy texture while increasing the good keto fats.

SPICY AVOCADO TUNA SALAD

FOR THE DRESSING

IN a bowl, combine the cilantro, olive oil, lemon zest and juice, paprika, salt, and pepper.

FOR THE SPICY TUNA

IN a serving bowl, toss together the tuna, avocados, cucumber, jalapeño, and red onion.

DRIZZLE the dressing over the top of the salad and serve.

NUTRITIONAL INFO (PER SERVING)
CALORIES 606, **FAT** 46.2 g, **PROTEIN** 38.2 g, **CARBS** 13.1 g, **FIBER** 8.6 g

---

MAKES 4 SERVINGS

~~~

DRESSING

¼ cup minced fresh cilantro

3 tablespoons extra-virgin olive oil

1 teaspoon grated lemon zest

2 tablespoons lemon juice

½ teaspoon smoked paprika

½ teaspoon salt

¼ teaspoon black pepper

SPICY TUNA

5 (5-ounce) cans tuna in water, drained

2 avocados, diced

1 cucumber, diced

1 fresh jalapeño pepper, diced

½ cup diced red onion

Bone broth is important when you are doing the keto diet because it contains tons of minerals and provides the electrolytes you need. I make it a point to drink a cup a day with a dab of butter and an extra sprinkle of salt on top. The amount of bone broth you end up with will vary depending on the size of your pressure cooker and how much liquid it can hold.

PRESSURE COOKER BONE BROTH

MAKES 15 CUPS

~~~

PREHEAT the oven to 400°F.

PLACE all the bones on a large baking sheet and roast for 30 minutes, until dark brown.

TRANSFER the bones to the pressure cooker. Add the onion, celery, vinegar, rosemary, salt, and enough water to reach the fill line of the cooker. Select the soup button, set the pressure to low, and increase the time setting to 120 minutes.

AFTER cooking, let the cooker naturally release the pressure. Strain the broth into a large bowl and discard the solids. Let the broth cool.

STORE in a covered container in the refrigerator for up to 4 days, or in the freezer for up to 4 months. Be sure to leave a little extra room at the top of the container to allow for expansion as the broth freezes.

- 2 to 4 pounds raw chicken or beef bones
- 1 onion, trimmed but left whole
- 2 stalks celery
- 2 tablespoons apple cider vinegar
- 2 sprigs fresh rosemary
- 1 tablespoon pink Himalayan salt

NUTRITIONAL INFO (PER 1 CUP)
CALORIES 34, **FAT** 1 g, **PROTEIN** 1.5 g, **CARBS** 4.9 g, **FIBER** 0.8 g

BROTH VS. STOCK

Many people are confused about the difference between stocks and broths. Broths are lighter and are traditionally made by simmering poultry, meat, or seafood in water—often with a few herbs or spices—and straining the liquid through a fine-mesh sieve.

Stocks are richer. They are made by simmering the bones from poultry, meat, or seafood in water, along with herbs or spices, for many hours, which pulls all the tasty flavor and healthy collagen from the bones. The longer you cook the bones, the richer the resulting stock.

Bone broth, despite its name, is actually richer than stock. It's generally made just like stock, using bones, but it's cooked for a much longer time—24 hours and sometimes longer, though you can speed that process up by using a pressure cooker. I like homemade best, but it's fine to use packaged broth or stock in a pinch.

Chicken stock is a fantastic base for so many recipes, and homemade always tastes the best. Making stock is a great way to make use of chicken bones. The next time you make dinner with bone-in chicken, save the bones in a zip-top plastic bag in the freezer. When you accumulate 2 to 4 pounds, it's a good day to make stock.

STOVETOP CHICKEN STOCK

COMBINE 20 cups water and all the ingredients in a large soup pot. Bring to a boil over high heat, lower the heat, and simmer for at least 6 hours or up to 12 hours. Skim off any foam that forms during the first couple hours of cooking. Stir occasionally and add water as needed; the water should cover the bones completely. Strain the stock into a large bowl and discard the solids. Let the stock cool.

STORE the cooled stock in a covered container in the refrigerator for up to 4 days, or in the freezer for up to 4 months. Be sure to leave a little extra room at the top of the container to allow for expansion as the stock freezes.

NOTE: *Roasted bones create an even richer, deeper flavor. Save any bones left over from your meals and roast in a 400°F oven for 15 minutes, until they become a dark brown, then use in the recipe. Be sure to also save any vegetable trimmings or scraps for stock. Simply toss them into the pot along with the other ingredients. It's a great way to use the parts you would normally throw away.*

MAKES 20 CUPS

∿∿∿

- 2 to 4 pounds raw or roasted chicken bones
- 1 onion, peel on, trimmed and chopped into large chunks
- 2 stalks celery, coarsely chopped
- 2 tablespoons apple cider vinegar
- 1 tablespoon pink Himalayan salt
- 2 sprigs fresh rosemary

NUTRITIONAL INFO (PER 1 CUP)
CALORIES 8, **FAT** 0.1, **PROTEIN** 1 g, **CARBS** 0.9 g, **FIBER** 0.2 g

This is the soup I use to boost my immune system when I'm feeling tired or not quite well. It also kills two birds with one stone: It's a hearty vegetable soup and it makes extra vegetable broth that you can enjoy later. I call for a full tablespoon of salt because it will help keep you hydrated. Some people like to control the amount of salt they ingest, so it's fine if you hold off adding the salt until the end, and your guests can add whatever amount makes them happy.

OLD-FASHIONED VEGETABLE SOUP

IN a large soup pot, mix together all the ingredients (add the salt after cooking if you prefer).

ADD 4 to 5 quarts water, leaving 2 inches at the top of the pot. Bring to a boil over medium-high heat. Lower the heat to medium-low and simmer until the vegetables are tender, about 2 hours. Stir occasionally and add more water if needed.

THIS soup is very brothy. I like to reserve about two-thirds (about 10 cups) of the liquid to refrigerate in covered containers (or freeze) to use later as vegetable broth. The remaining soup will be thick and hearty.

STORE the soup in a covered container in the refrigerator for up to 4 days, or in the freezer for up to 4 months.

NUTRITIONAL INFO (PER SERVING)
CALORIES 76, **FAT** 4.8 g, **PROTEIN** 2.2 g, **CARBS** 7.3 g, **FIBER** 1.9 g

MAKES 6 SERVINGS, PLUS 15 CUPS ADDITIONAL VEGETABLE BROTH

~~~~~

- 8 ounces radishes, trimmed and quartered
- 8 ounces mushrooms, quartered
- 2 baby bok choy, chopped
- 1 medium onion, chopped
- 1 medium leek, chopped, white and pale-green parts only
- ¼ cup lemon juice
- 2 tablespoons coconut oil
- 1 tablespoon ground turmeric
- 1 tablespoon salt
- 2 teaspoons grated lemon zest
- 2 teaspoons minced fresh garlic
- 1 teaspoon minced fresh ginger
- 1 teaspoon black pepper

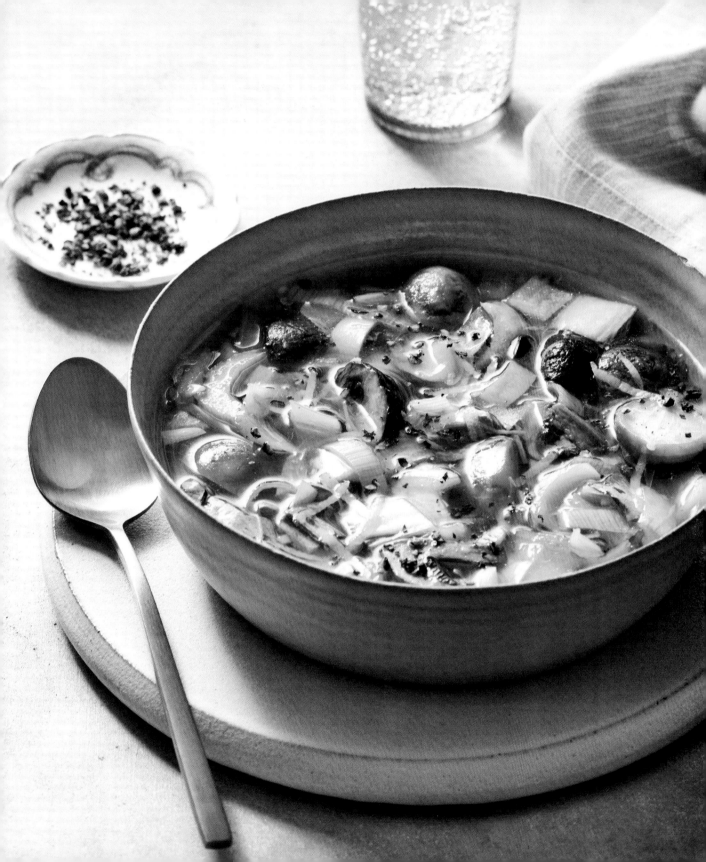

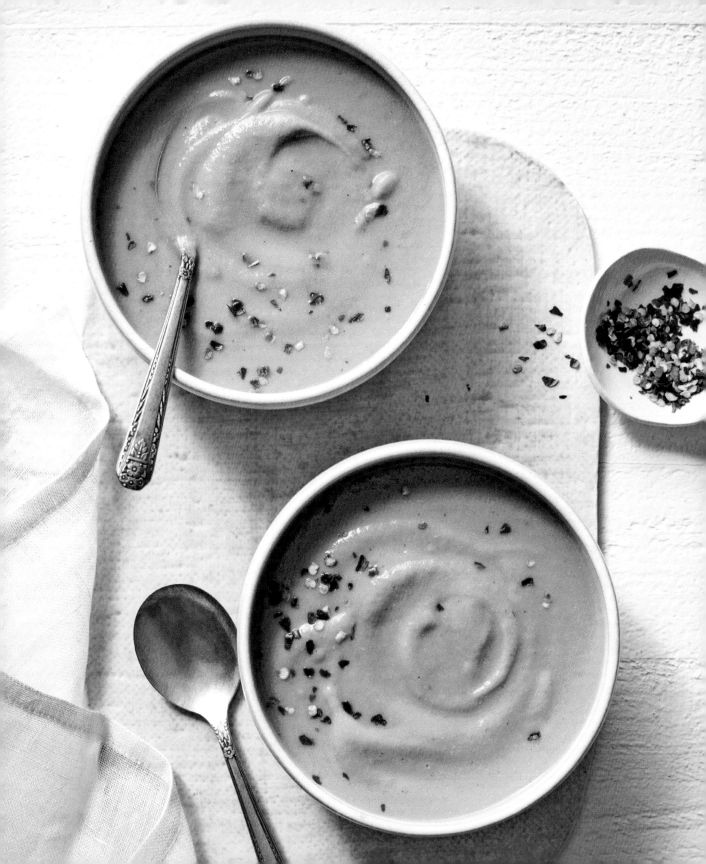

I usually make this with canned pumpkin because it's fast and easy, but you can also use fresh pumpkin. Simply cut 3 pounds fresh pumpkin into chunks and cook it along with the radishes until tender. Serve with a warm Keto Bagel (page 196) topped with everything-but-the-bagel seasoning.

THAI COCONUT PUMPKIN SOUP

HEAT the oil in a soup pot over medium heat. Add the radishes and onion and cook until the onion is translucent and the radishes have softened, 6 to 7 minutes. Add the bone broth, bring to a boil, lower the heat, and simmer until the radishes are tender, about 20 minutes.

ADD the pumpkin puree, garlic, curry powder, and nutmeg. Cover and cook until the soup is heated through, another 5 minutes. Remove from the heat and let cool for about 5 minutes.

PUREE the soup in a blender (or with an immersion blender right in the pot) until smooth. Return the soup to the pot and add the coconut milk and red pepper flakes, if using. Stir to combine and cook over medium heat, stirring occasionally, until heated through.

NUTRITIONAL INFO (PER SERVING)
CALORIES 98, **FAT** 2.6 g, **PROTEIN** 3.4 g, **CARBS** 16.6 g, **FIBER** 4.6 g

MAKES 8 SERVINGS

∿∿∿

1 tablespoon extra-virgin olive oil

8 ounces radishes, trimmed and quartered

1 medium onion, chopped

3 cups Pressure Cooker Bone Broth (page 65) or store-bought bone broth

1 (15-ounce) can pumpkin puree

2 teaspoons minced garlic

2 teaspoons curry powder

½ teaspoon ground nutmeg

1 (10-ounce) can full-fat coconut milk

1 teaspoon crushed red pepper flakes, optional

You will be shocked at how much this tastes like real potato soup. It might even feel like cheating, but there is no need for guilt here. Even if you don't like raw radishes, I strongly suggest you try them, because when they are cooked they take on a creamy texture that is very potato-like. You can use a (10- or 12-ounce) bag of frozen riced cauliflower instead of florets to save time.

TASTES JUST LIKE POTATO SOUP

PREHEAT the oven to 400°F.

SPREAD out the cauliflower florets and radishes on a baking sheet, drizzle with the olive oil, and season with the salt and pepper. Roast for 30 to 35 minutes, until tender.

TRANSFER the roasted vegetables to a soup pot. Stir in the broth, garlic, cream cheese, and paprika and bring to a boil over medium-high heat. Lower the heat to medium-low and simmer for 10 minutes. Remove from the heat and let cool for about 5 minutes.

PUREE the soup in a blender (or with an immersion blender right in the pot) until smooth. Return the soup to the soup pot, pour in the coconut milk, and cook over low heat until heated through, 4 to 5 minutes.

SERVE with cheese and bacon on the side, if you like.

NUTRITIONAL INFO (PER SERVING)
CALORIES 255, **FAT** 20.8 g, **PROTEIN** 8.8 g, **CARBS** 11 g, **FIBER** 3.3 g

MAKES 4 SERVINGS

~~~~

- 1 head cauliflower, cut into florets
- 4 ounces radishes, trimmed and quartered
- 2 tablespoons extra-virgin olive oil
- 1 teaspoon salt
- ½ teaspoon black pepper
- 4 cups Stovetop Chicken Stock (page 67) or store-bought vegetable broth (or broth from Old-Fashioned Vegetable Soup, page 68)
- 3 tablespoons minced garlic
- 2 ounces cream cheese
- 1 teaspoon paprika
- ½ cup full-fat coconut milk

OPTIONAL GARNISHES
shredded cheddar cheese and bacon bits

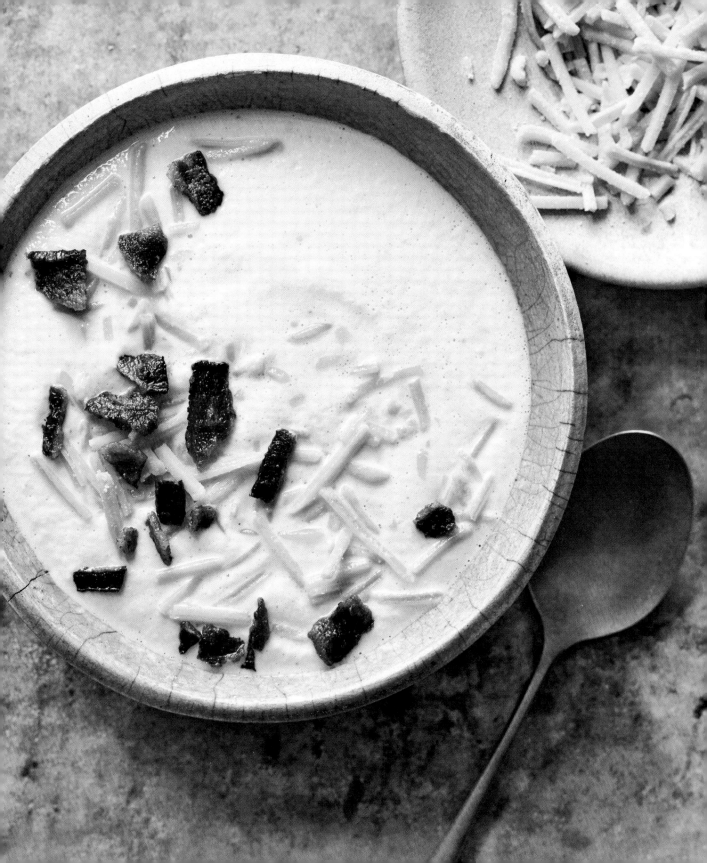

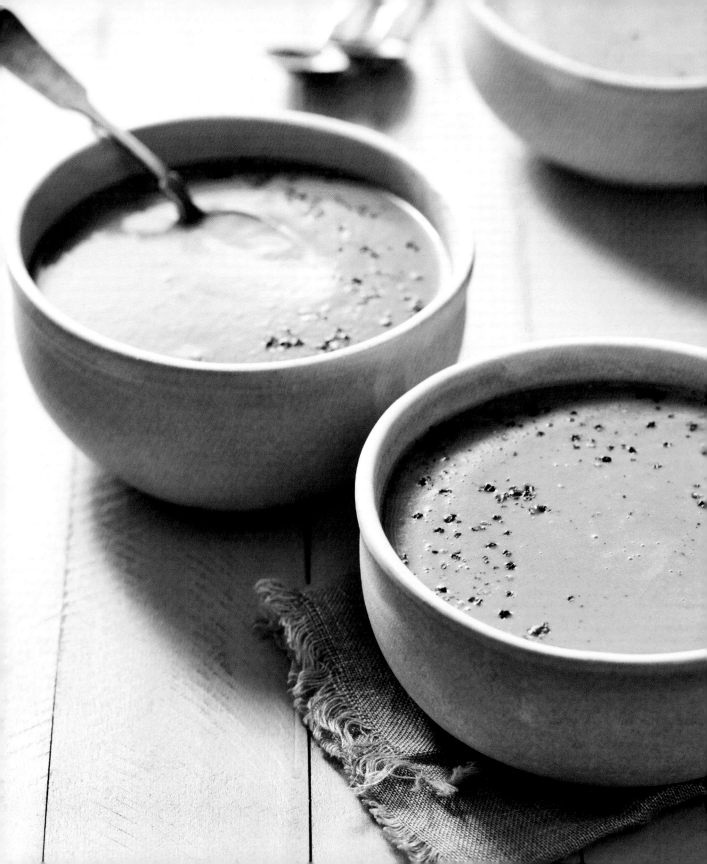

Loaded with healthy fats that will keep you full for a long time, this incredibly creamy soup is wonderful with a warm toasted Keto Bagel (page 196) or a Low-Carb Biscuit (page 184) making a complete meal. Tomatoes tend to be higher in carbs than other vegetables so this recipe should be a rare treat.

CREAMY ROASTED TOMATO SOUP

MAKES 6 SERVINGS

IN a large soup pot over medium heat, heat the olive oil. Add the onion and cook, stirring, until translucent, 4 to 5 minutes. Add the garlic and cook, stirring, for 1 minute. Add 2 cups water, the tomatoes, and the stock and bring to a boil. Lower the heat to a simmer and continue to cook for another 20 to 30 minutes, until the tomatoes break down and the flavors develop.

ADD the cream, cream cheese, salt, and pepper and cook, stirring, for another 5 minutes. Remove from the heat and let cool for 5 minutes. Puree until smooth in a blender or with an immersion blender right in the pot.

- 2 tablespoons extra-virgin olive oil
- 1 medium onion, diced
- 2 teaspoons minced garlic
- 1 (28-ounce) can fire-roasted tomatoes, diced or crushed
- 2 cups Stovetop Chicken Stock (page 67) or store-bought chicken broth
- 1 cup heavy cream
- 4 ounces cream cheese
- 2 teaspoons salt
- 1 teaspoon black pepper

NUTRITIONAL INFO (PER SERVING)
CALORIES 287, **FAT** 25.8 g, **PROTEIN** 3.6 g, **CARBS** 10.7 g, **FIBER** 2.3 g

I am a newfound radish lover. And I discovered that you don't always need to eat them raw. When they are cooked, they get tender like a potato and their flavor mellows so you can add other flavors—in this case sausage—and make them the star of the meal.

KETO ITALIAN SOUP

MAKES 8 SERVINGS

~~~

IN large pot over medium heat, cook the sausage, breaking it up with a wooden spoon, until completely browned. Add the broth, radishes, onion, and garlic and cook, stirring, until the radishes are tender, about 20 minutes. Add the cream and kale and continue to cook until the kale is tender, about 10 minutes.

SPOON into bowls and serve immediately.

- 1 pound bulk mild Italian sausage
- 4 cups Stovetop Chicken Stock (page 67) or store-bought vegetable broth (or broth from Old-Fashioned Vegetable Soup, page 68)
- 1 pound radishes, trimmed and diced
- 1 medium onion, diced
- 2 teaspoons minced garlic
- 1/3 cup heavy cream
- 2 to 3 cups bite-size pieces kale

NUTRITIONAL INFO (PER SERVING)
CALORIES 192, **FAT** 14.8 g, **PROTEIN** 7.1 g, **CARBS** 8.9 g, **FIBER** 2.6 g

VARIATION
Substitute cauliflower for the radishes, which will also be very delicious.

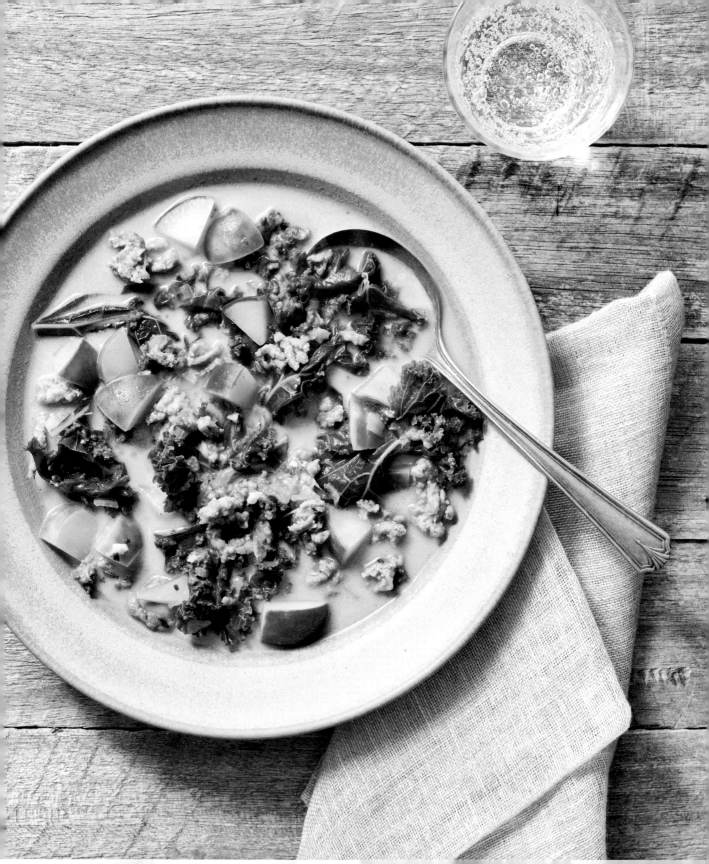

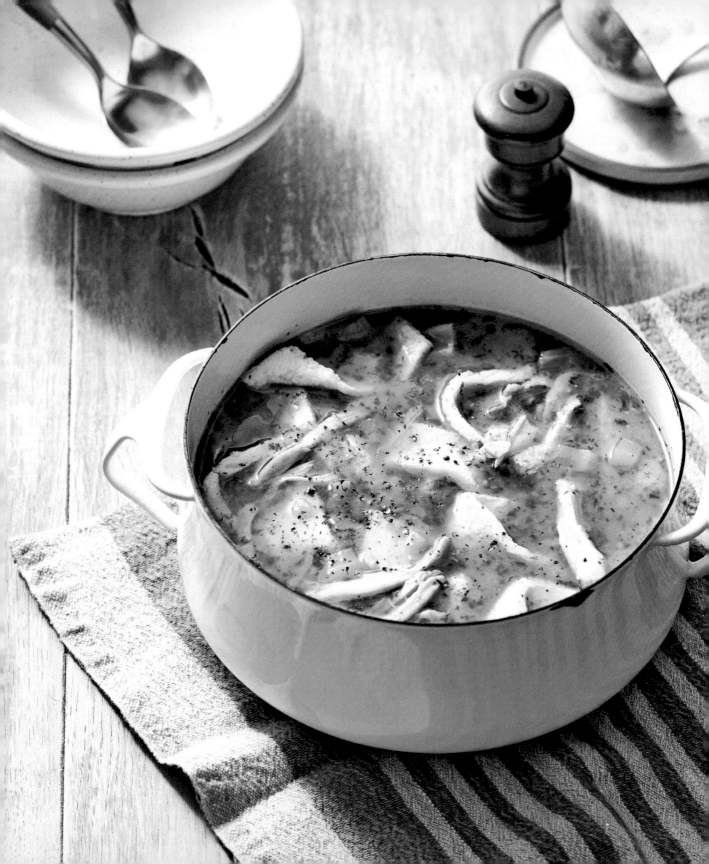

The dumplings in this recipe are really special. Served in a warm soup, they take on the flavors of the stock, with a texture you may remember from childhood. The trick to successful keto dumplings is to roll them out thick and put them in the pot just before serving because they don't need a long time to cook. This recipe is well-loved by my non-keto friends too!

CHICKEN AND DUMPLING SOUP

FOR THE SOUP

IN a large Dutch oven, heat the olive oil over medium-high heat. Season the chicken all over with salt and pepper. Add the chicken to the pot and brown for 4 to 6 minutes per side. Transfer the chicken to a plate and set aside.

ADD the celery, onion, garlic, and thyme to the pot and cook, stirring, until soft, 5 to 7 minutes. Add 4 cups water, the stock, melted butter, and bay leaves and stir to combine. Add the chicken back, bring the mixture to a boil, lower the heat to medium-low, and simmer for 20 minutes, until the chicken is cooked through.

TRANSFER the chicken to a cutting board and shred the meat from the bones with a fork. Discard the bones (or save to make Stovetop Chicken Stock, page 67). Add the shredded chicken back to the Dutch oven and cook for another 10 minutes, until heated through.

FOR THE DUMPLINGS

HAVE a silicone mat ready. Place the mozzarella in a microwave-safe bowl and heat in the microwave oven until fully melted, about 1½ minutes. Add the coconut flour, baking powder, xanthan gum, and egg yolks and mix together. It will make a stiff dough.

TRANSFER the dough to the silicone mat and knead until smooth. Using a rolling pin, roll out the dough to the edges of the mat, or until it's ½ inch thick. Using a pizza cutter or a sharp knife, gently

(continued)

MAKES 6 SERVINGS

~~~

SOUP

1 tablespoon extra-virgin olive oil

2 pounds bone-in skin-on chicken thighs

Salt and black pepper

4 stalks celery, chopped

1 medium onion, chopped

3 cloves garlic, chopped

2 tablespoons fresh thyme (or 2 teaspoons dried thyme)

2 cups Stovetop Chicken Stock (page 67) or store-bought chicken broth

8 tablespoons butter, melted

2 bay leaves

DUMPLINGS

2 cups shredded part-skim low-moisture mozzarella cheese

½ cup coconut flour

½ teaspoon baking powder

½ teaspoon xanthan gum

3 large egg yolks

cut strips of dough about 1 inch wide. Sprinkle the strips with a bit of coconut flour so they don't stick to one another.

JUST before serving, carefully add the strips to the soup, 4 or 5 at a time so they won't stick to each other, and cook very gently for 2 to 3 minutes. Serve immediately.

NUTRITIONAL INFO (PER SERVING)
CALORIES 576, **FAT** 36.3 g, **PROTEIN** 45.7 g, **CARBS** 15.9 g, **FIBER** 4.5 g

VARIATION
For a creamier soup, stir in ½ cup heavy cream after the dumplings have cooked.

NOTE: *To get this on the dinner table even faster, buy a cooked rotisserie chicken at the grocery store and shred the meat from the bones. Make the soup as above, starting with cooking the vegetables. Increase the chicken stock to 4 cups, add the shredded chicken, and cook until heated through. Then continue following the recipe to cook the dumplings.*

Mushroom lovers, this is for you. It's rich and creamy and it tastes even better the next day.

CREAMY MUSHROOM SOUP

MELT the butter in a large soup pot over medium heat. Add the onion and cook, stirring, until translucent, 4 to 5 minutes. Add the mushrooms and thyme and cook, stirring, until the mushrooms are soft and tender, 5 to 6 minutes. Add the stock and bring to a boil. Lower the heat to low and let simmer for about 10 minutes, until the flavors develop.

TRANSFER ½ cup of the broth to a blender and add the cream cheese. Blend on high until pureed. Pour the cream cheese mixture back into the soup pot and add the cream, salt, and pepper. Simmer, stirring, for another 5 minutes, until heated through.

JUST before serving, add the parsley.

NUTRITIONAL INFO (PER SERVING)
CALORIES 379, **FAT** 33 g, **PROTEIN** 11.2 g, **CARBS** 14.4 g, **FIBER** 2.9 g

> **VARIATION**
> If you would like to lower the fat content, omit the cream cheese and add 1 teaspoon xanthan gum when you add the cream. This will give the soup its creamy consistency without adding fat.

MAKES 4 SERVINGS

~~~

- 2 tablespoons butter
- 1 medium onion, diced
- 1½ pounds button or cremini mushrooms, trimmed and sliced
- 1 tablespoon minced fresh thyme
- 5 cups Stovetop Chicken Stock (page 67) or store-bought chicken broth
- 4 ounces cream cheese
- ¾ cup heavy cream
- 1 teaspoon salt
- ½ teaspoon black pepper
- 3 tablespoons minced fresh parsley

Here's a terrific taco soup via three different methods: stovetop, slow cooker, or Instant Pot or pressure cooker. A pressure cooker is so speedy it allows you to get a delicious dinner on the table in no time at all! But the slow cooker can be cooking away while you are off on a hike or relaxing and reading a book. There is a cooking method for every lifestyle, including traditionalists who prefer the stovetop. If you like, add sliced jalapeños or avocado in addition to all the other toppings.

EASY TACO SOUP—THREE WAYS

MAKES 6 SERVINGS

~~~~

2 pounds ground pork or beef (or a mix of both)

4 cups Stovetop Chicken Stock (page 67) or store-bought chicken broth

2 (10-ounce) cans Ro*Tel mild diced tomatoes and green chilies

2 (8-ounce) packages cream cheese

2 tablespoons Taco Seasoning (page 235)

OPTIONAL TOPPINGS

shredded cheese, chopped fresh cilantro, sliced black olives, sour cream, sliced radishes

STOVETOP METHOD

IN a large skillet over medium-high heat, cook the ground beef, breaking it up with a wooden spoon as it cooks, until browned. Drain the excess oil and set aside the beef.

ADD the stock, Ro*Tel, cream cheese, and taco seasoning to a large pot over medium-high heat and mix together. Add the browned beef and mix. Bring to a boil, lower the heat to medium-low, and simmer until cooked through, 15 to 20 minutes.

SLOW COOKER METHOD

IN a large skillet over medium-high heat, cook the ground beef, breaking it up with a wooden spoon as it cooks, until browned. Drain the excess oil and set aside the beef.

ADD the stock, Ro*Tel, cream cheese, and taco seasoning to the slow cooker and mix together. Add the browned beef and mix. Cover and cook on low for 4 hours or on high for 2½ hours.

INSTANT POT OR PRESSURE COOKER METHOD

COOK the beef using the sauté setting of the cooker, breaking the meat up with a wooden spoon as it cooks, until browned. Add the stock, Ro*Tel, cream cheese, and taco seasoning and mix together. Pressure cook for 5 minutes using the soup setting. Use the quick release.

TO serve, spoon the soup into bowls and serve with optional toppings on the side.

NUTRITIONAL INFO (PER SERVING)
CALORIES 560, **FAT** 41.5 g, **PROTEIN** 36.4 g, **CARBS** 9.5 g, **FIBER** 0.4 g

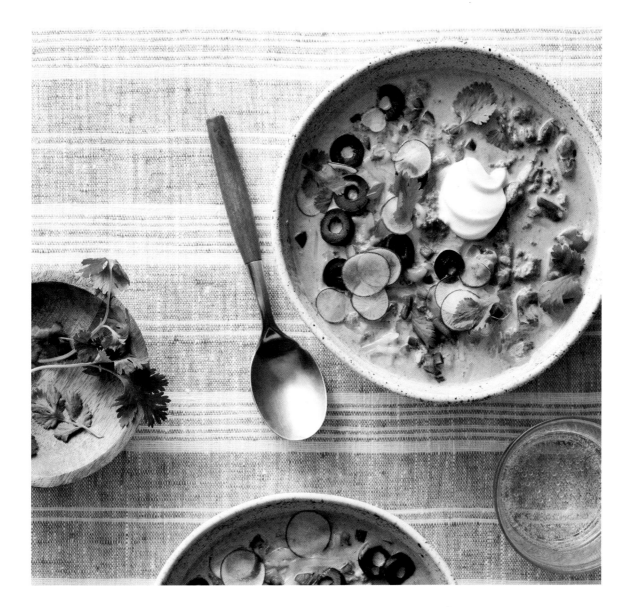

4
MAIN DISHES

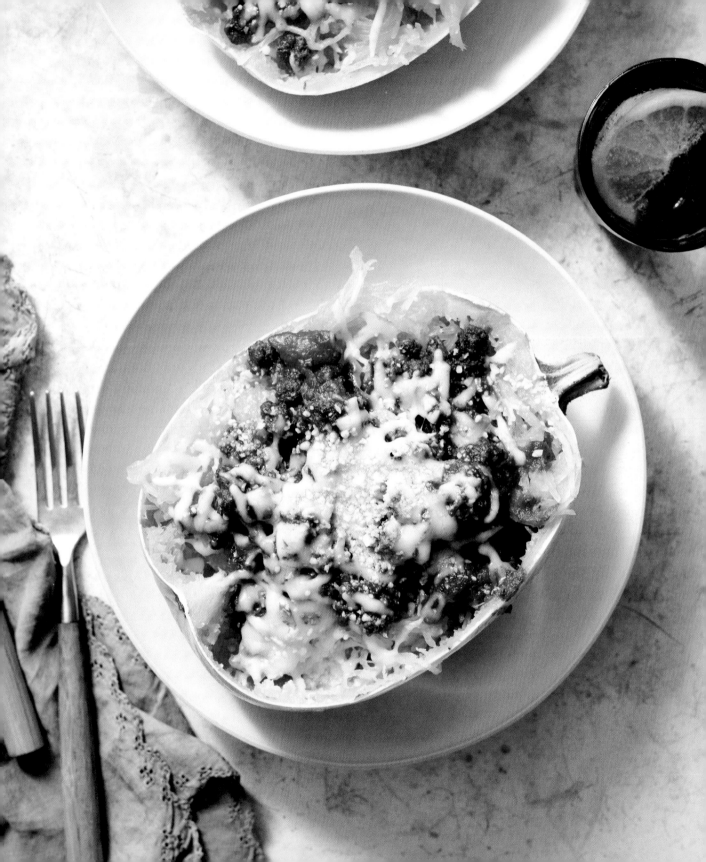

It's fine to use a jarred marinara sauce in this dish to save time, but be sure to read the label closely because many prepared sauces have added sugar in them, which you do not want.

ITALIAN SPAGHETTI-SQUASH BOWLS

PREHEAT the oven to 350°F. Line a baking sheet with parchment paper or a silicone mat.

CUT the spaghetti squash in half, scoop out the seeds, and place it into an Instant Pot or pressure cooker. Add 1 cup water, press manual, and pressure cook on high for 15 minutes. Use the quick release, transfer the squash to a large bowl, and cool slightly. (If you don't have an Instant Pot or pressure cooker, cut the squash in half, scoop out the seeds, coat with 1 teaspoon olive oil, and sprinkle with salt and pepper. Place cut side down on a baking pan and bake at 400°F for 40 minutes, until tender.)

USE a fork to scrape the spaghettilike strands from the squash into a large bowl, then add the butter. Reserve the squash "bowls," placing them on the prepared baking sheet.

IN a large skillet over medium-high heat, cook the ground beef, breaking the meat up with a wooden spoon, until browned. Add the marinara, garlic, salt, and pepper and cook, stirring. Add the spaghetti squash and mix together until combined.

SPOON the ground beef mixture equally between the two squash bowls. Top with the mozzarella and Parmesan. Bake for 5 to 10 minutes, until the cheese melts and becomes golden brown.

NUTRITIONAL INFO (PER SERVING)
CALORIES 288, **FAT** 16.3 g, **PROTEIN** 26.3 g, **CARBS** 8.9 g, **FIBER** 2.1 g

MAKES 2 SERVINGS

~~~

1 small spaghetti squash

2 tablespoons butter

½ pound ground beef

½ cup Homemade Marinara Sauce (page 236)

½ teaspoon minced garlic

¼ teaspoon salt

¼ teaspoon black pepper

1 cup shredded part-skim low-moisture mozzarella cheese

2 tablespoons grated Parmesan cheese

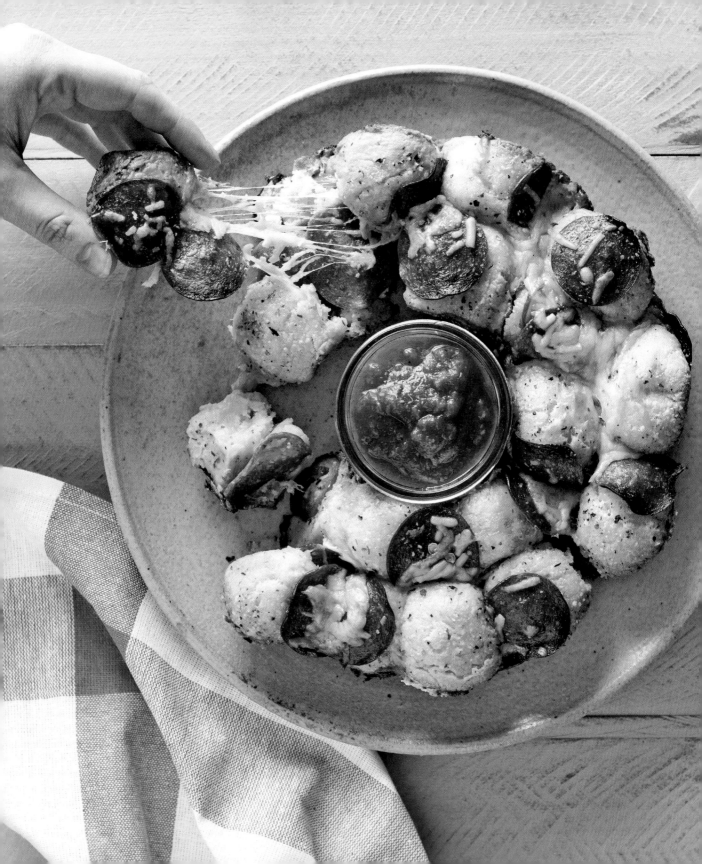

If you are having a bunch of friends over to watch the football game, they'll love snacking on this newfangled version of pizza. Rolling the balls of dough in grated Parmesan is the secret to being able to easily pull apart the bread. Serve with a small bowl of Homemade Italian Marinara Sauce (page 236) for lots of dipping fun.

PULL-APART PIZZA BREAD

MAKES 12 SERVINGS

PREHEAT the oven to 350°F. Spray a Bundt pan with cooking spray. Have a silicone mat ready. Mix together the Parmesan and rosemary in a small bowl and set aside.

IN a medium bowl, mix the almond flour with the baking powder until fully combined.

IN a microwave-safe bowl, heat the mozzarella cheese and cream cheese in the microwave oven until melted, about 1 minute. Add the almond flour mixture and the eggs and mix until it forms a sticky ball. Transfer to the silicone mat.

SPRINKLE the dough with some additional Parmesan to keep it from being too sticky. Cut the dough into 32 pieces. Roll each piece of dough into a ball and then roll them in the Parmesan mixture. Place 16 of the dough balls in the prepared Bundt pan. Sprinkle half of the shredded cheddar over the dough balls. Layer half of the sliced pepperoni over the cheese, and top with jalapeños, if using. Repeat the layering with the rest of the dough balls, cheddar, pepperoni, and jalapeños, if using.

BAKE for 25 minutes, until golden brown. Let cool for 5 minutes. Invert the pan onto a plate and serve.

- ½ cup grated Parmesan cheese, plus more as needed
- 1 tablespoon chopped fresh rosemary
- 1½ cups blanched almond flour
- 1 tablespoon baking powder
- 2½ cups shredded part-skim low-moisture mozzarella cheese
- 2 ounces cream cheese
- 3 large eggs, beaten
- ½ cup shredded mild cheddar cheese
- ½ cup sliced pepperoni
- Sliced fresh jalapeño peppers, optional

NUTRITIONAL INFO (PER SERVING)
CALORIES 216, **FAT** 16.3 g, **PROTEIN** 12.1 g, **CARBS** 7.3 g, **FIBER** 1.9 g

Roasted radishes are the secret ingredient that you mix with eggs and cheese to create a delicious stand-in for pasta. I call for mascarpone cheese because it has a higher fat content than cream cheese, but either will work. You can serve this meal with a side salad and Homemade Ranch Salad Dressing (page 231) to help get your fats up even more!

AMAZING KETO LASAGNA

MAKES 8 SERVINGS

~~~~

PREHEAT the oven to 400°F. Line a baking sheet with parchment paper or a silicone mat. Spray the bottom of an 11½- by 15-inch baking pan with cooking spray.

FOR THE RADISH NOODLES

IN a bowl, mix together the radishes, olive oil, and a pinch of salt. Spread the radishes out evenly on the prepared baking sheet and roast for 20 to 25 minutes, until tender. Lower the oven temperature to 350°F.

COMBINE the radishes, eggs, mascarpone, and mozzarella in a blender and pulse until pureed. Reline the baking sheet with parchment paper. Spread the radish mixture evenly onto the parchment paper and bake for 10 to 12 minutes, until soft. Let cool.

USING a sharp knife, cut the baked radish mixture into long slices, each about 2 inches wide. Set aside.

TO ASSEMBLE THE LASAGNA

IN a medium skillet over medium-high heat, cook the ground beef in the oil, breaking it up with a wooden spoon, until browned. Season with salt and pepper to taste.

IN a bowl, combine the ricotta cheese with the eggs, parsley, oregano, basil, Italian seasoning, and garlic powder and mix until fully combined.

(continued)

RADISH NOODLES

1 cup quartered trimmed radishes

1 tablespoon extra-virgin olive oil

Pinch of salt

3 large eggs

4 ounces mascarpone cheese or cream cheese

½ cup shredded part-skim low-moisture mozzarella cheese

LASAGNA

1½ pounds ground beef

2 teaspoons extra-virgin olive oil

Salt and black pepper

1 cup whole-milk ricotta cheese

3 large eggs

1 tablespoon dried parsley

1 teaspoon dried oregano

1 teaspoon dried basil

1 teaspoon dried Italian seasoning

(ingredients continued)

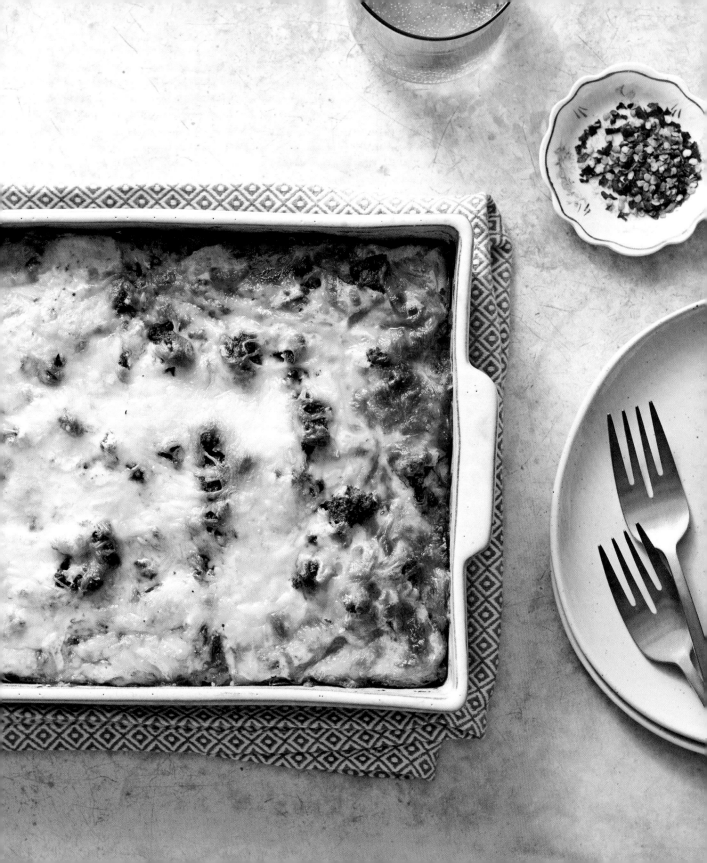

SPOON a little marinara sauce on the bottom of the baking dish. Overlap about 3 of the radish noodles until the sauce is completely covered. Dollop spoonfuls of the ricotta mixture over the noodles, then some of the beef, and then a layer of marinara. Top with some shredded mozzarella. Repeat two or three times, or until you run out of ingredients, making sure to finish with a layer of mozzarella.

BAKE for about 40 minutes, until the cheese starts to brown and the lasagna is bubbly. Let cool for about 10 minutes before serving.

½ teaspoon garlic powder

1 cup Homemade Marinara Sauce (page 236)

1½ cups shredded part-skim low-moisture mozzarella cheese

NUTRITIONAL INFO (PER SERVING)
CALORIES 317, **FAT** 23.9 g, **PROTEIN** 17.8 g, **CARBS** 7.9 g, **FIBER** 1.1 g

VARIATION
You can replace the radishes in the noodle recipe with 1 cup packed raw kale or spinach.

With a treat that is so filling, it's best to serve it with a light side salad to avoid feeling too full. The recipe makes a wonderful dough that you can pack with almost any of your favorite meats.

KETO CALZONES

PREHEAT the oven to 350°F. Line two baking sheets with parchment paper or silicone mats.

IN a small skillet, cook the ground beef over medium-high heat, breaking it up with a wooden spoon, until browned. Add the cheddar and marinara and mix until combined. Set aside.

IN a microwave-safe bowl, mix together the mozzarella and parsley until combined. Heat in the microwave oven until it melts, about 1 minute. Add the almond flour and egg and mix until just combined.

TRANSFER the dough to one prepared baking sheet and knead until it comes together. Place a sheet of parchment paper on top of the dough and use a rolling pin to roll out the dough to an approximate 6- by 8-inch rectangle about ¼ inch thick. Cut the dough into 12 (2-inch) squares.

PLACE about 1 tablespoon of the beef mixture in the center of one dough square, making sure to keep the edges free of sauce (otherwise the dough won't stick together properly). Fold the dough over to form a triangle and press the edges together with a fork to seal them.

REPEAT to make 12 calzones, placing each on the second prepared baking sheet.

BAKE for 15 to 20 minutes, until golden brown.

SERVE hot.

MAKES 12 CALZONES (6 SERVINGS)

~~~~

8 ounces ground beef

⅔ cup shredded cheddar or Colby cheese

3 tablespoons Homemade Marinara Sauce (page 236) or store-bought low-sugar marinara

1¾ cups shredded part-skim low-moisture mozzarella cheese

1 tablespoon chopped fresh parsley

¾ cup blanched almond flour

1 large egg

NUTRITIONAL INFO (PER SERVING)
CALORIES 173, **FAT** 17.3 g, **PROTEIN** 20.2 g, **CARBS** 5.5 g, **FIBER** 1.6 g

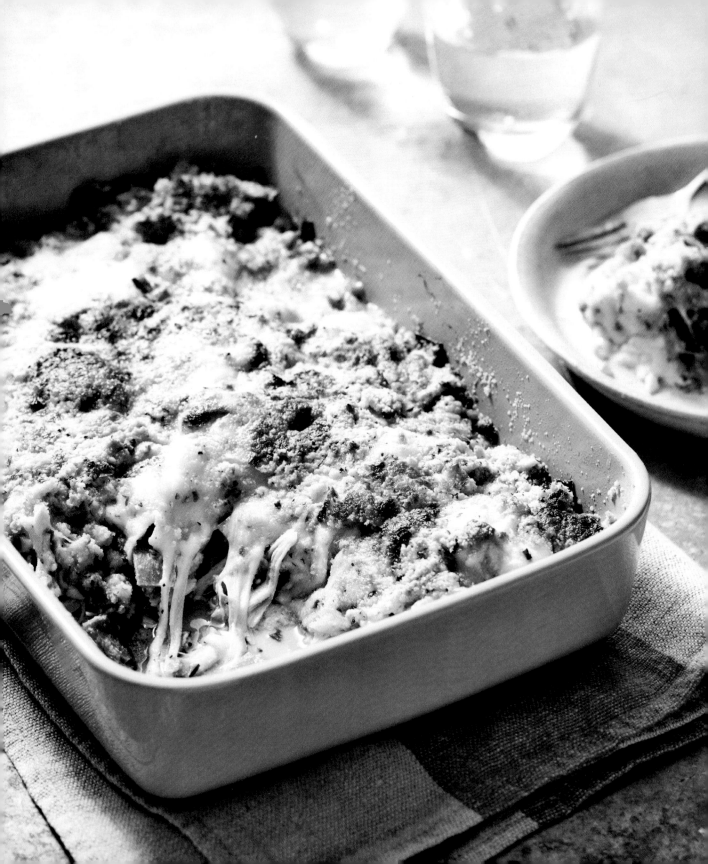

This crowd-pleasing casserole borrows the wonderful flavors of the classic French dish for a great main course, perfect for a potluck or to serve during a Sunday football game.

CHICKEN CORDON BLEU CASSEROLE

PREHEAT the oven to 375°F. Spray a 9- by 13-inch baking dish with cooking spray.

IN a large bowl, mix together the chicken, sour cream, heavy cream, mustard, ½ teaspoon salt, and ¼ teaspoon pepper.

TRANSFER the chicken mixture to the prepared baking dish, spreading it evenly. Top with the ham and cream cheese pieces. Cover the top with the slices of Swiss cheese.

IN a bowl, mix together the almond flour, Italian seasoning, ½ teaspoon salt, and ¼ teaspoon pepper. Sprinkle the almond flour mixture over the top of the Swiss cheese. Top with the pieces of butter.

BAKE for 30 minutes, until bubbly. If you prefer a browned topping, place the casserole under the broiler for about 2 minutes.

NUTRITIONAL INFO (PER SERVING)
CALORIES 513, **FAT** 39.8 g, **PROTEIN** 33.2 g, **CARBS** 6.9 g, **FIBER** 1.5 g

MAKES 8 SERVINGS

~~~

2 skinless boneless chicken breasts (6 ounces), cooked and shredded

½ cup sour cream

¼ cup heavy cream

2 teaspoons Dijon mustard

Salt and black pepper

8 ounces sliced ham, chopped

4 ounces cream cheese, cut into pieces

8 ounces sliced Swiss cheese

1 cup blanched almond flour

1 tablespoon dried Italian seasoning

8 tablespoons butter, cut into pieces

The keto community has really fallen in love with this recipe, maybe because it's so easy to make and has lots of healthy fats, or maybe because it tastes so good it's practically addictive. It's versatile too: Serve it as a dip or make it the main attraction at dinner along with a side of zucchini noodles or mashed cauliflower. You can make this recipe on the stovetop, but it's also great when made in the pressure cooker. I've included instructions for both.

CRACK CHICKEN

MAKES 10 SERVINGS

PRESSURE COOKER METHOD

POUR the bone broth into the bottom of an Instant Pot or pressure cooker. Add the chicken and cream cheese and sprinkle with the ranch seasoning.

SET the pressure cooker on high to cook for 12 minutes if using chicken breasts or 10 minutes if using tenders. Use a quick release.

TRANSFER the chicken to a cutting board and shred using two forks. Return the shredded chicken to the pressure cooker. Add the cheddar and crumbled bacon and mix everything together.

PLACE the lid back on the pressure cooker (but don't turn it on) and let sit for about 5 minutes, until the cheese has melted and formed a thick sauce. Stir everything together to combine.

STOVETOP METHOD

IN a deep skillet over medium-high heat, cook the chicken in the oil until browned and fully cooked, 8 to 10 minutes per side. Transfer the chicken to a cutting board and shred using two forks. Return the shredded chicken to the skillet.

ADD the bone broth, cream cheese, and ranch seasoning, stir, and cook until the cream cheese has melted and formed a thick sauce. Add the cheddar cheese and crumbled bacon and mix everything together.

- 1 cup Pressure Cooker Bone Broth (page 65), store-bought bone broth, or water
- 2 pounds boneless skinless chicken breasts or chicken tenders
- 2 tablespoons olive oil (if cooking on the stovetop)
- 12 ounces cream cheese, cut into large cubes
- ¼ cup Homemade Dry Ranch Seasoning (page 230)
- ½ cup shredded cheddar cheese, plus more for serving
- 8 ounces sugar-free nitrite-free bacon, cooked and crumbled, plus more for serving
- ¼ cup sliced green onions, optional
- ¼ cup Frank's RedHot Buffalo Wings Sauce, optional

TOP with additional shredded cheese and crumbled bacon, plus green onions and hot sauce, if using, and serve.

NOTE: *If you are doing strict keto, please note that commercially made ranch seasoning packets contain maltodextrin, an ingredient I try to stay away from. The recipe for Homemade Dry Ranch Seasoning (page 230) includes instructions for making it in bulk so you'll always have it in the pantry ready to use.*

NUTRITIONAL INFO (PER SERVING)
CALORIES 571, **FAT** 40.2 g, **PROTEIN** 40.2 g, **CARBS** 13.9 g, **FIBER** 0.1 g

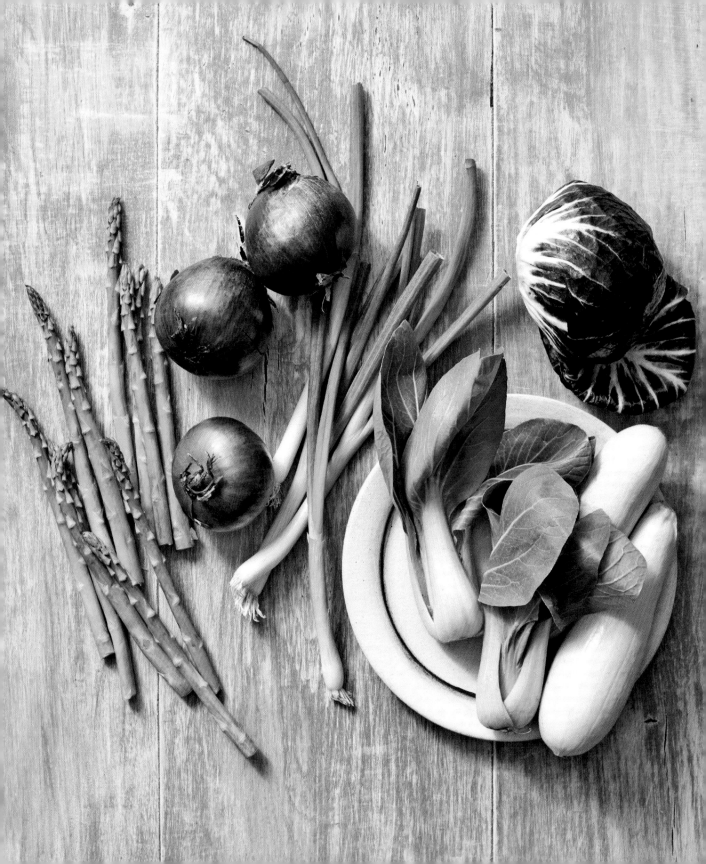

"Zoodles" is zucchini that has been cut into noodles. If you enjoy them as much as I do, I strongly suggest investing in a vegetable spiralizer, which makes it easy to cut the zucchini very thin. You can buy precut zoodles, but you'll pay a much higher price—and who wants that? If you don't have a spiralizer, you can also use a mandoline or even a vegetable peeler, but it will take longer to cut the zoodles. It's worth every bit of effort though.

CHICKEN ALFREDO WITH ZOODLES

MAKES 6 SERVINGS

FOR THE ALFREDO SAUCE

IN a medium saucepan, mix ¼ cup water with the cream cheese, Parmesan, butter, cream, and garlic. Cook over medium heat, stirring, until the cheese is melted and the ingredients are fully combined. Add the spinach and mix to completely cover in the sauce. Let cook until the spinach is tender, 1 to 2 minutes. Add the chicken and cook until heated through.

FOR THE ZOODLES

CUT the zucchini into zoodles using a spiralizer. Alternatively, you can cut the zucchini into thin strips with a mandoline or vegetable peeler.

IN a saucepan set over high heat, boil 1 cup water. Add the zoodles, lower the heat to a simmer, cover the pan, and steam until tender, 5 to 8 minutes. Drain.

TO serve, place a small amount of zoodles on a plate or in a bowl and top with the alfredo sauce.

ALFREDO SAUCE

8 ounces cream cheese

¾ cup grated Parmesan cheese

8 tablespoons butter

¼ cup heavy cream

1 teaspoon minced garlic

2 handfuls fresh spinach

12 ounces shredded cooked chicken

ZOODLES

5 or 6 medium zucchini

NUTRITIONAL INFO (PER SERVING)
CALORIES 444, **FAT** 36.6 g, **PROTEIN** 25.7 g, **CARBS** 3.5 g, **FIBER** 0.4 g

This makes an excellent weeknight dinner because it cooks up very quickly. This classic Italian dish with sun-dried tomatoes and spinach includes heavy cream, a keto-friendly fat. Serve with cauliflower mash or cauliflower rice for a complete meal that the whole family will love. Lemon-pepper seasoning can be found in the spice section of your grocery store.

CREAMY TUSCAN CHICKEN

SEASON the chicken on all sides with the lemon-pepper seasoning.

IN a large skillet, warm the olive oil over medium-high heat. Add the chicken and cook, turning once, until cooked all the way through, 8 to 12 minutes per side. Transfer to a plate and set aside.

TO the same skillet, add the onion and cook, stirring occasionally, until translucent, 3 to 5 minutes. Add the stock and garlic and cook, using a spoon to scrape up any brown bits that may have stuck to the bottom of the pan. Pour in the cream and add the Parmesan cheese, garlic powder, and Italian seasoning. Stir until the cheese melts and the ingredients are incorporated.

LOWER the heat to medium-low and add the spinach and sun-dried tomatoes, letting the spinach wilt and the sun-dried tomatoes heat through for 3 to 5 minutes. Add the chicken to the mixture and serve.

NUTRITIONAL INFO (PER SERVING)
CALORIES 440, **FAT** 33.7 g, **PROTEIN** 24.1 g, **CARBS** 12.7 g, **FIBER** 2.6 g

MAKES 4 SERVINGS

~~~

- 2 skinless boneless chicken breasts (about 10 ounces total)
- 3 tablespoons lemon-pepper seasoning
- 2 tablespoons extra-virgin olive oil
- ½ onion, diced
- ½ cup Stovetop Chicken Stock (page 67) or store-bought chicken broth
- 5 tablespoons minced garlic
- 1 cup heavy cream
- ½ cup grated Parmesan cheese
- 1 teaspoon garlic powder
- 1 teaspoon dried Italian seasoning
- 3 cups baby spinach
- 5 ounces sun-dried tomatoes, cut into julienne strips

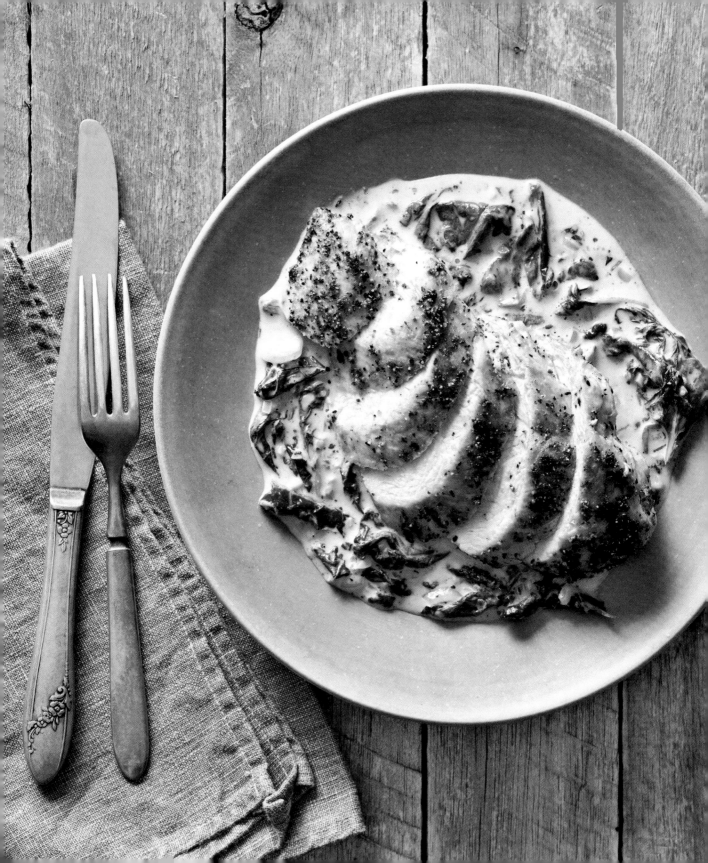

Buy a rotisserie chicken on the way home from work and you can easily make this dish and have this casserole in the oven in less than half an hour. Salsa verde is a green Mexican sauce made with finely chopped onions, garlic, cilantro, parsley, and hot peppers. It comes in jars and you can find it in the Mexican foods section of most grocery stores. It adds a nice punch of flavor to just about any dish.

SALSA VERDE CHICKEN CASSEROLE

PREHEAT the oven to 350°F. Have a 9- by 13-inch baking dish ready.

IN a medium bowl, combine the cauliflower, 1 cup of the shredded cheese, the salsa verde, sour cream, cream cheese, cilantro, and garlic. Add the shredded chicken and the Ro*Tel, if using, and mix together. Spoon the mixture into the baking dish and spread evenly. Sprinkle the remaining 1 cup shredded cheese over the top.

BAKE for 30 minutes, until heated through and the topping starts to brown. Serve hot.

NOTE: *Use frozen cauliflower florets if you'd like to save a little time. Just add them per the recipe and check to be sure they're cooked through before serving. If they're not, return to the oven and bake for 10 more minutes.*

MAKES 12 SERVINGS

~~~

- 1 pound cauliflower (see Note), cut into small florets
- 2 cups shredded Mexican cheese blend or Monterey Jack cheese
- 1½ cups salsa verde
- 1 cup sour cream
- 8 ounces cream cheese, softened
- ¼ cup minced fresh cilantro
- ½ teaspoon minced garlic
- 2 cups shredded cooked chicken or turkey
- 1 (10-ounce) can Ro*Tel mild diced tomatoes and green chilies, drained, optional

NUTRITIONAL INFO (PER SERVING)
CALORIES 299, **FAT** 19 g, **PROTEIN** 15.3 g, **CARBS** 19.6 g, **FIBER** 1.3 g

Any cut of chicken will work here, but if you are looking to increase your fat intake, use bone-in chicken thighs, drumsticks, or wings instead of chicken breasts.

GARLIC-CILANTRO GRILLED CHICKEN

DIVIDE the chicken between two large zip-top plastic bags.

IN the bowl of a food processor or blender, combine the cilantro, garlic, olive oil, lime juice, sweetener, salt, and pepper and mix on high until nearly smooth. Pour half of the marinade into each zip-top bag, remove as much air as possible, and seal. Marinate in the refrigerator for at least 1 hour or up to 24 hours.

PREPARE a gas or charcoal grill for cooking (you can use a stovetop grill pan as well).

REMOVE the chicken from the marinade, shaking off any excess. Grill until cooked through, 5 to 7 minutes on each side. (Watch closely. Cooking times may vary depending on the heat of your grill).

NUTRITIONAL INFO (PER SERVING)
CALORIES 234, **FAT** 8.7 g, **PROTEIN** 34.4 g, **CARBS** 3.7 g, **FIBER** 0.3 g

MAKES 6 SERVINGS

2 pounds boneless chicken breasts

¾ cup chopped fresh cilantro

3 tablespoons minced garlic

2 tablespoons extra-virgin olive oil

Juice of 3 limes

½ teaspoon monkfruit sweetener

½ teaspoon salt

¼ teaspoon black pepper

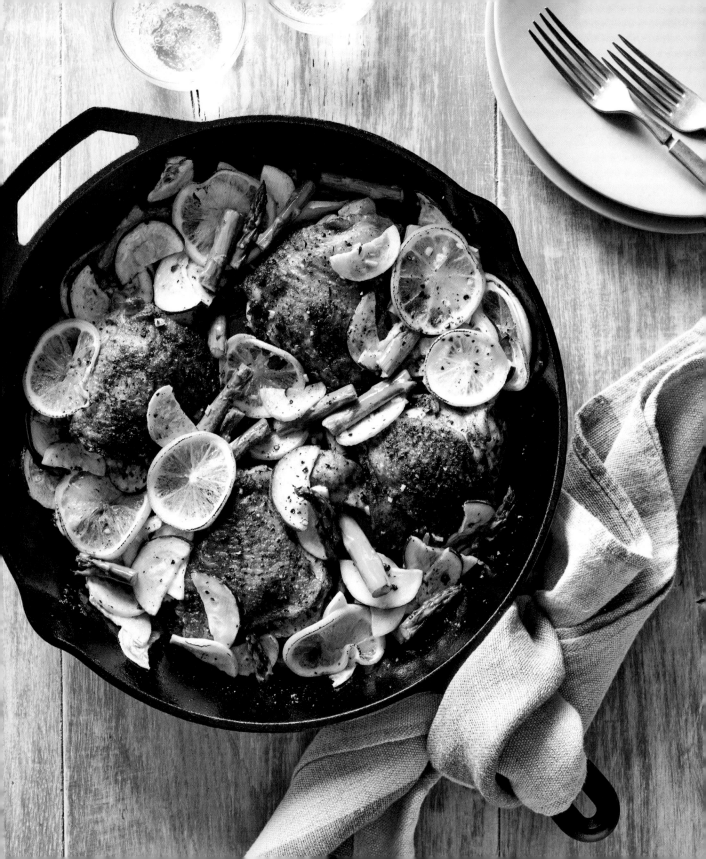

I love cooking in a cast-iron skillet. Not only does it cook food more evenly than other pans, it is nonstick when seasoned properly, and—bonus!—you get a little extra iron in your diet. In this recipe, you start cooking the chicken on the stovetop and then finish in the oven, and the cast-iron skillet can do both!

LEMON-GARLIC CHICKEN

PREHEAT the oven to 375°F.

IN a large bowl, mix together the lemon juice, garlic, oregano, and salt and pepper to taste. Add the chicken and mix, making sure all sides of the chicken are covered.

IN a large cast-iron pan over medium-high heat, heat the oil until it just starts to smoke. Shake off any excess liquid from the chicken, add to the pan, and cook until browned, about 4 minutes on each side.

ADD the asparagus, zucchini, and lemon slices. Transfer the pan to the oven and bake for 30 minutes, until the chicken is cooked through.

NUTRITIONAL INFO (PER SERVING)
CALORIES 235, **FAT** 15.1 g, **PROTEIN** 18.9 g, **CARBS** 7.4 g, **FIBER** 2 g

MAKES 4 SERVINGS

Juice of 1 lemon

3 cloves garlic, minced

2 teaspoons dried oregano

Salt and black pepper

4 (4-ounce) bone-in chicken thighs

3 tablespoons extra-virgin olive oil

½ pound asparagus, trimmed and cut into 2-inch pieces

1 zucchini, cut in half lengthwise and sliced into half-moons

1 lemon, sliced

Using an air fryer to cook the chicken results in crispy wings without all the bad fat you get from frying in oil. Serve them with a side of steamed veggies or a salad for a full meal, or bring them to a party as a yummy appetizer. If you don't have an air fryer, I've also included instructions to roast them in the oven.

BUFFALO CHICKEN WINGS

AIR FRYER METHOD

PREHEAT the air fryer to 400°F.

SEASON the chicken wings with the salt and pepper. Place the wings in the air fryer basket and bake for 25 minutes, flipping them halfway through the cook time, until cooked through.

OVEN METHOD

PREHEAT the oven to 400°F. Place a wire rack on a baking sheet.

SEASON the chicken wings with the salt and pepper. Place the wings on the prepared baking sheet and bake for 45 to 50 minutes, turning once after 25 minutes, until cooked through.

TO SERVE

IN a large bowl, mix together the hot sauce, butter, pepper, and garlic powder. Toss the hot chicken wings with the sauce mixture. Serve the wings with celery sticks, ranch dressing, or blue cheese dressing if you like.

NUTRITIONAL INFO (PER SERVING)
CALORIES 122, **FAT** 12 g, **PROTEIN** 2.4 g, **CARBS** 2.1 g, **FIBER** 0.5 g

MAKES 4 SERVINGS

~~~

- 2 pounds chicken wings or drumettes
- 1 teaspoon salt
- 1 teaspoon black pepper
- ½ cup Frank's RedHot hot sauce
- 4 tablespoons butter, melted
- ¼ teaspoon black pepper
- ½ teaspoon garlic powder

OPTIONAL ACCOMPANIMENTS
celery sticks, blue cheese dressing, ranch dressing

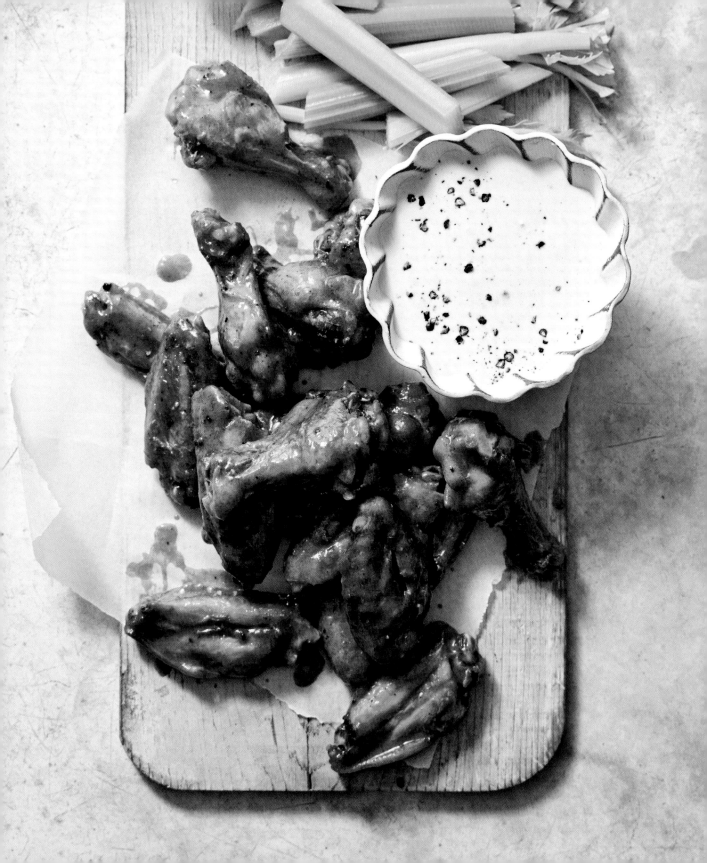

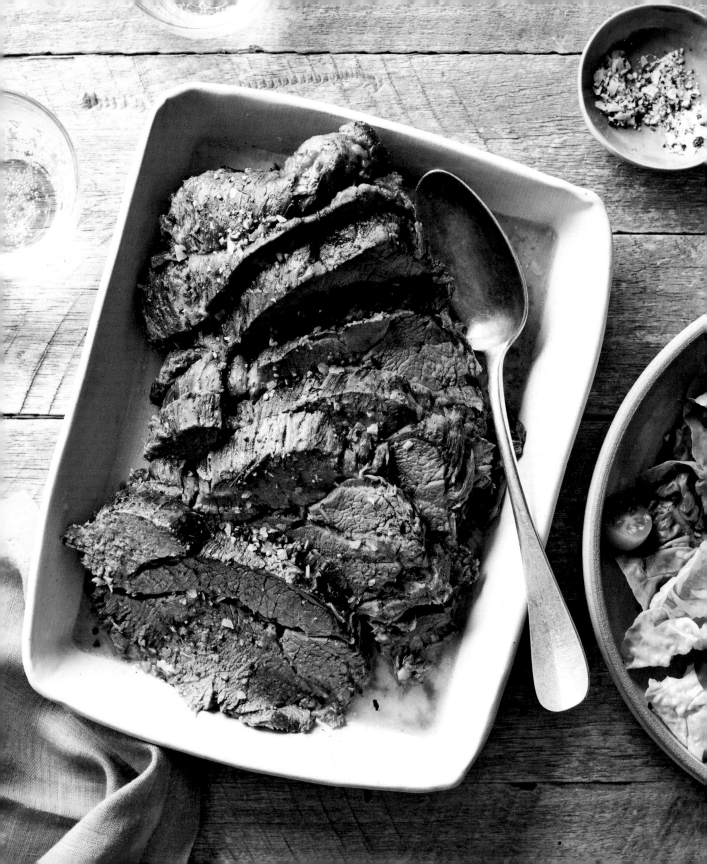

A chuck roast always tastes best when you cook it low and slow. Once I found this recipe and realized how many different meals I could make with it, following the keto diet became so much easier. Cut the roast into small pieces and mix it with cauliflower rice, add it to your morning scrambled eggs, or put it between two slices of Savory Keto Bread (page 189). If you buy a 32-ounce jar of pickles, you should have enough juice for this recipe. (I buy 64-ounce jars at my local warehouse club so I always have pickle juice on hand.) Serve with Cauliflower-Creamed Spinach (page 168) and Parmesan Zucchini Crisps (page 176) for a substantial meal impressive enough for company.

SLOW-COOKER DILL-PICKLE POT ROAST

MAKES 8 SERVINGS

~~~

4 to 5 pounds beef chuck roast

3 to 4 cups dill pickle juice

1 or 2 sprigs fresh rosemary or thyme, or 1 to 2 tablespoons Montreal steak seasoning

SPRAY the inside of a slow cooker with cooking spray or line the cooker with a slow cooker liner.

ADD the roast to the slow cooker and pour the pickle juice over the top. If the juice doesn't come at least halfway up the side of the beef, add water until it does. Place the sprigs of rosemary or thyme on top of the beef roast, or sprinkle the Montreal steak seasoning over the top.

SET the slow cooker on low, cover, and cook for at least 8 hours, until the roast is completely tender. Start the cooking in the morning and it will be ready right when everyone gets home for dinner.

STORE any leftover pot roast in a covered container in the refrigerator for up to 4 days or in the freezer for up to 4 months.

NUTRITIONAL INFO (PER SERVING)
CALORIES 370, **FAT** 14.4 g, **PROTEIN** 55.8 g, **CARBS** 0.9 g, **FIBER** 0.4g

This is an excellent dish served with riced cauliflower or in lettuce wraps. Normally bulgogi is made with rib eye steak, but flank steak is a money-saving option and I use it all the time. Be sure to cut the flank steak against the grain.

KOREAN BULGOGI FLANK STEAK

PLACE the flank steak in the freezer for about 20 minutes prior to slicing it to make it easier to cut. Cut the meat against the grain into ¼-inch-thick slices. Place in a shallow baking dish.

IN a bowl, combine the onion, coconut aminos, stock, sweetener, garlic, ginger, sesame oil, and vinegar. Pour over the beef, making sure that it's covered with the marinade. Cover and marinate in the refrigerator for at least 3 hours or up to overnight. The longer you marinate, the more tender the steak.

WHEN ready to cook, heat the oil in a skillet over medium heat. Add the steak slices and cook until done to your liking, 1 to 2 minutes per side. You may need to cook them in batches to avoid overcrowding. Sprinkle with the green onions and sesame seeds and serve.

NUTRITIONAL INFO (PER SERVING)
CALORIES 395, **FAT** 16.7, **PROTEIN** 51.2 g, **CARBS** 10.1 g, **FIBER** 0.7 g

MAKES 4 SERVINGS

2 pounds flank steak

½ onion, diced

5 tablespoons coconut aminos

¼ cup Stovetop Chicken Stock (page 67), store-bought chicken broth, or water

3 tablespoons Sukrin Gold brown sugar sweetener

2 tablespoons minced garlic

½ teaspoon minced fresh ginger

1 tablespoon sesame oil

1 tablespoon rice vinegar

1 teaspoon extra-virgin olive oil

2 green onions, sliced

Sesame seeds

Pair the pork belly with a side of grilled vegetables or salad. It also tastes great with a spoonful of Blueberry Sauce (page 243) on top. Pork belly is loaded with fat and is very rich, so a small serving goes a long way.

OVEN-ROASTED PORK BELLY

PREHEAT the oven to 400°F. Have a baking dish ready.

RUB the pork belly on all sides with the olive oil. Sprinkle the salt, pepper, and sweetener, if using, all over the pork belly.

PLACE the pork belly in the baking dish fat side up and roast for 30 minutes. Turn over the belly, lower the heat to 300°F, and continue to roast for another hour, until meltingly tender. Cut into 8 pieces and serve.

NUTRITIONAL INFO (PER SERVING)
CALORIES 324, **FAT** 33.6 g, **PROTEIN** 5.3 g, **CARBS** 0 g, **FIBER** 0 g

MAKES 8 SERVINGS

~~~

- 1 pound slab pork belly
- 2 tablespoons extra-virgin olive oil
- 2 teaspoons salt
- 2 teaspoons black pepper
- 2 teaspoons monkfruit sweetener, optional

Serve the steak on its own and it conforms perfectly to the keto plan. But feel free to serve it with a side salad if you feel you need a little more.

GARLIC-BUTTER RIB EYE STEAK STRIPS

MAKES 4 SERVINGS

~~~

2 (8-ounce) rib eye steaks

PLACE the steaks in the freezer for about 20 minutes prior to slicing to make them easier to cut. Cut the meat against the grain into ½-inch-thick slices. Place in a shallow baking dish.

MARINADE

⅔ cup coconut aminos

⅔ cup extra-virgin olive oil

3 tablespoons lemon juice

2 tablespoons sriracha or other hot sauce of choice

1 teaspoon grated lemon zest

FOR THE MARINADE

COMBINE all the marinade ingredients in a bowl. Pour over the steaks, making sure that all the steak is covered. Cover and marinate in the refrigerator for at least 30 minutes or up to 24 hours. The longer you marinate, the more tender the steak.

FOR THE SPINACH, STEAK, AND SAUCE

PLACE the spinach in a large skillet set over medium heat, drizzle with the olive oil, and toss until fully coated. Cook until the spinach has wilted, 3 to 4 minutes. Transfer the spinach to a bowl and set aside.

SPINACH AND SAUCE

1 pound fresh spinach

2 tablespoons extra-virgin olive oil

3 tablespoons butter

¼ cup minced garlic

¼ cup Pressure Cooker Bone Broth (page 65) or store-bought bone broth

¼ cup fresh thyme leaves

¼ cup chopped fresh chives

2 teaspoons lemon juice

¼ teaspoon red pepper flakes, crushed or ground

1 teaspoon salt

½ teaspoon black pepper

TO the same skillet, add 2 tablespoons of the butter and melt over medium-high heat. Add the steak strips and cook for 1 minute on each side or to your liking. You may need to cook them in batches to avoid overcrowding. Transfer the steak to a bowl and set aside.

TO the same skillet, add the remaining 1 tablespoon butter, the garlic, broth, thyme leaves, chives, lemon juice, and red pepper. Bring to a boil, lower the heat to a simmer, and reduce the sauce, stirring constantly, until thick, 2 to 3 minutes. Season with the salt and pepper.

RETURN the steak to the pan, arrange the spinach around the steak, and cook until heated through. Serve warm.

NUTRITIONAL INFO (PER SERVING)
CALORIES 410, **FAT** 34.8, **PROTEIN** 15 g, **CARBS** 16.6 g, **FIBER** 6.4 g

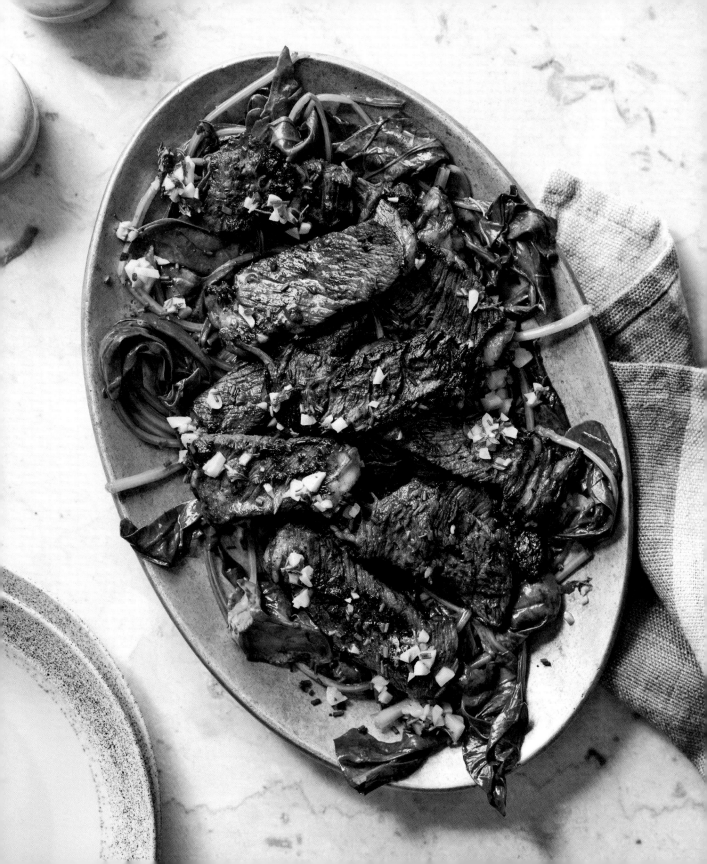

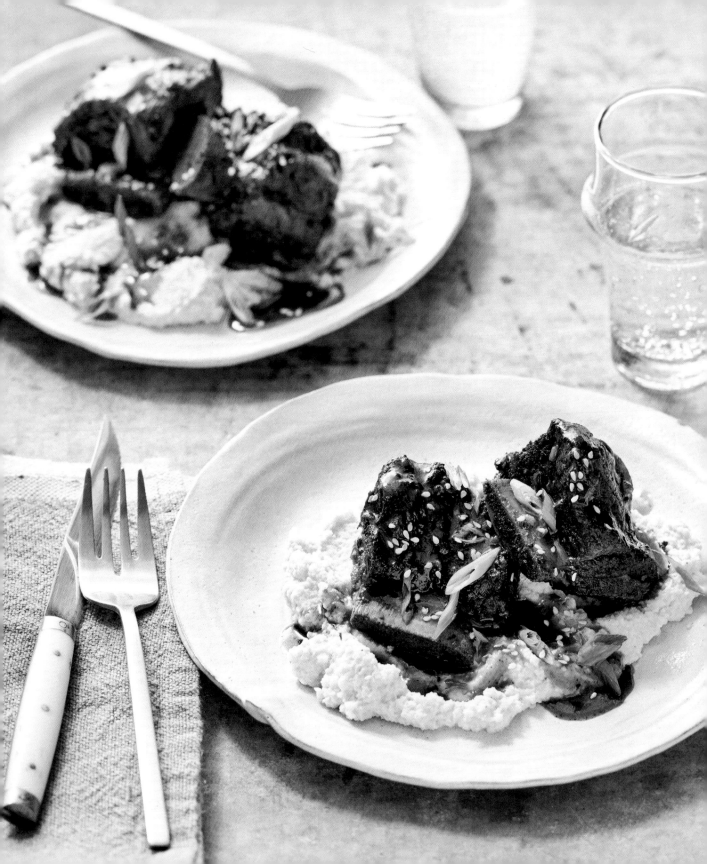

Don't expect any leftovers when you make these ribs—everyone will eat every bit. Spoon them over mashed cauliflower and add a side vegetable for a full meal. Here I give both grilling and pressure cooking instructions.

BRAISED BEEF SHORT RIBS

MAKES 4 SERVINGS

IN a large zip-top plastic bag, combine the short ribs and all the remaining ingredients. Seal and marinate in the refrigerator for at least 3 hours or up to overnight. The longer you marinate, the more tender the ribs.

GAS GRILL METHOD
PREHEAT a gas grill to 400°F. Remove the short ribs from the marinade, shaking off any excess. Grill the short ribs for 15 to 20 minutes, until brown and tender. The internal temperature should be 130°F for perfect tenderness.

INSTANT POT OR PRESSURE COOKER METHOD
ADD the short ribs and their marinade to an Instant Pot or pressure cooker and cook on high pressure for 45 minutes. It sounds like a long time, and they are good after 30 minutes, but they come out extremely tender if you cook them for the full 45 minutes.

NUTRITIONAL INFO (PER SERVING)
CALORIES 404, **FAT** 22.7 g, **PROTEIN** 47.1 g, **CARBS** 5.6 g, **FIBER** 0.5 g

2 pounds short ribs

¼ cup coconut aminos

¼ cup Stovetop Chicken Stock (page 67), store-bought chicken broth, or water

2 tablespoons sliced green onion

2 tablespoons Swerve confectioners' sweetener

1 tablespoon black pepper

2 teaspoons sesame oil

1 teaspoon minced garlic

1 teaspoon salt

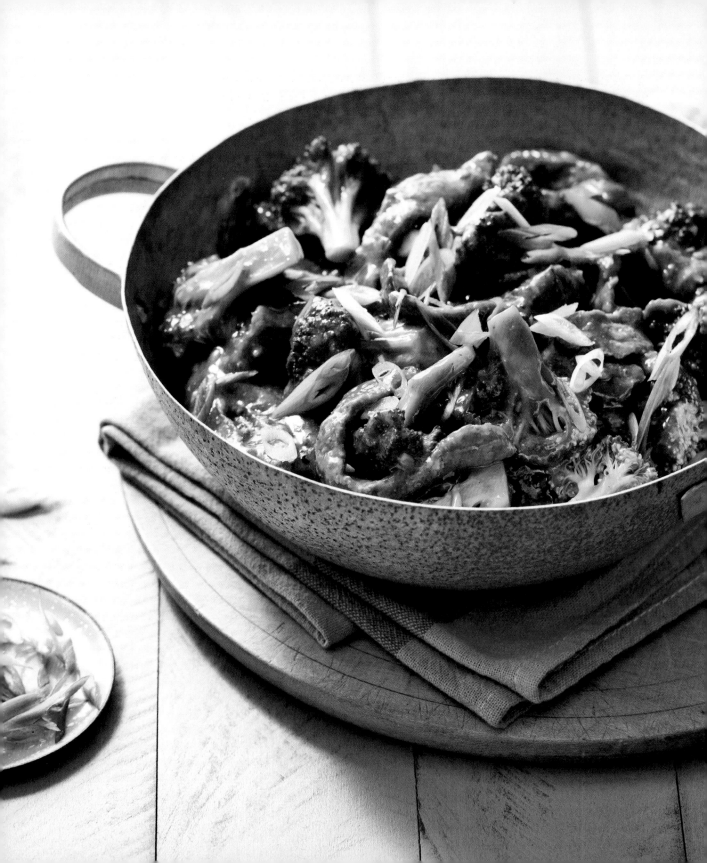

To make this recipe even easier, have the butcher slice the flank steak when you buy it. I think this goes very well with a cup of Old-Fashioned Vegetable Soup (page 68).

MONGOLIAN BEEF AND BROCCOLI

MAKES 4 SERVINGS

〜〜〜

1 pound flank steak

3 tablespoons extra-virgin olive oil

2 teaspoons minced garlic

1 teaspoon grated fresh ginger

½ cup Pressure Cooker Bone Broth (page 65), store-bought bone broth, or water

⅓ cup Sukrin Gold brown sugar sweetener

2 tablespoons coconut aminos

1 teaspoon xanthan gum

1 (12-ounce) bag frozen broccoli florets

¼ cup whey protein isolate

1 teaspoon salt

½ teaspoon black pepper

2 green onions, sliced

PLACE the flank steak in the freezer for about 20 minutes prior to slicing it to make it easier to cut.

IN a saucepan over medium heat, heat 2 tablespoons of the olive oil. Add the garlic and ginger and cook, stirring, for 1 minute. Lower the heat and add the broth, sweetener, and coconut aminos and simmer for 3 to 4 minutes. Sprinkle in the xanthan gum and mix well. Remove the sauce from the heat and set aside.

PLACE the frozen broccoli in a microwave-safe dish with ⅓ cup water and heat in the microwave oven on high for 5 minutes, until the broccoli is tender. Set aside.

IN a shallow dish, add the whey protein isolate. Remove the steak from the freezer and cut against the grain into ½-inch-thick slices. Season the slices with the salt and pepper. Dip each slice into the whey protein isolate and set aside on a plate.

IN a skillet over medium-high heat, heat the remaining 1 tablespoon olive oil. Add the steak slices and cook to your liking, 1 to 2 minutes on each side. Add the sauce and mix thoroughly. Add the broccoli and mix again.

GARNISH with green onions and serve warm.

NUTRITIONAL INFO (PER SERVING)
CALORIES 287, **FAT** 16.5 g, **PROTEIN** 28.3 g, **CARBS** 8.2 g, **FIBER** 3 g

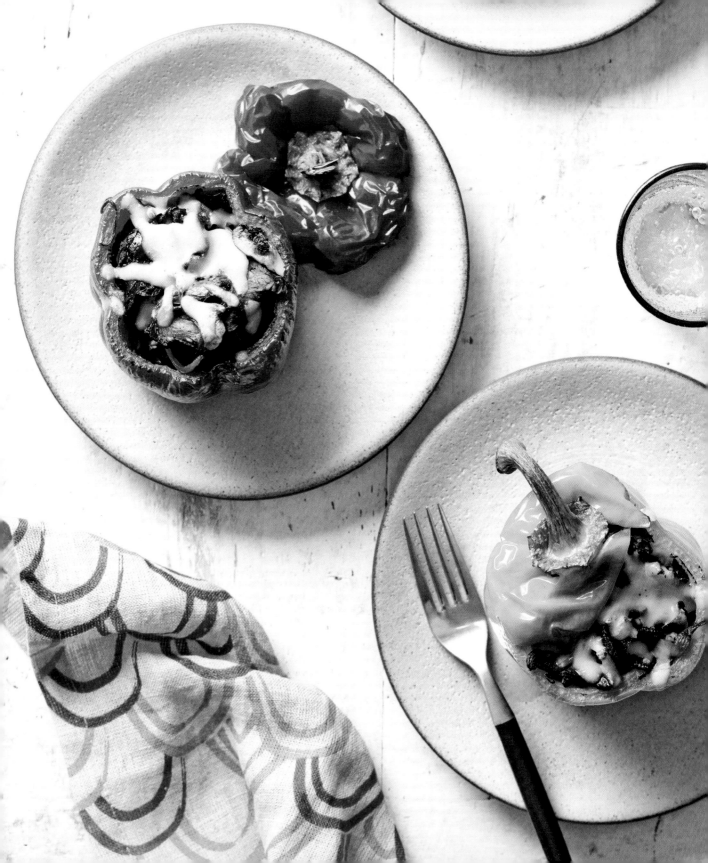

I love stuffed peppers and Philly cheesesteak, so I was thrilled when I created a way to combine them. Typically, the Philly cheesesteak is made with rib eye steak, but you can also make it with sirloin. To cut the thin slices of steak, freeze the meat for about an hour before you start slicing it. The meat will be solid enough to cut very thin slices, but not too frozen to cut easily. A sharp knife is a must. Don't forget to cut the meat against the grain. You can also ask your butcher to shave the steak, which will save you the effort.

PHILLY CHEESESTEAK STUFFED PEPPERS

MAKES 4 SERVINGS

PREHEAT the oven to 400°F.

IN a large skillet over medium-high heat, heat the oil. Add the onion and cook, stirring, for 1 minute. Add the steak, Worcestershire, parsley, salt, and pepper and continue to cook, stirring, for 3 to 4 minutes. Add the mushrooms and cook, stirring, for an additional 1 to 2 minutes, until the steak is done to your liking. Remove the pan from the heat and set aside.

CUT ½ inch off the top of each bell pepper. Remove the stem, seeds, and membranes. (If necessary, cut a tiny bit off the bottoms so they will stand up on their own.) Press 1 slice of provolone cheese into the cavity of each bell pepper, then spoon in one-fourth of the steak mixture.

PLACE the stuffed peppers on a rimmed baking sheet and bake for 40 minutes. Remove the pan from the oven and top the peppers with the shredded mozzarella. Return to the oven and continue to bake until the cheese is melted and bubbly, about 5 minutes. Serve hot.

- 1 tablespoon extra-virgin olive oil
- 1 onion, thinly sliced
- 1 pound rib eye steak, shaved or sliced very thinly
- 2 tablespoons Worcestershire sauce
- 1 tablespoon dried parsley
- ½ teaspoon salt
- ¼ teaspoon black pepper
- 4 ounces sliced mushrooms
- 4 large bell peppers
- 4 slices provolone cheese
- 4 ounces shredded part-skim low-moisture mozzarella cheese

NUTRITIONAL INFO (PER SERVING)
CALORIES 405, **FAT** 21.6 g, **PROTEIN** 34.8 g, **CARBS** 18.7 g, **FIBER** 4.2 g

The trick to this recipe is in the pork rinds, one of my favorite ingredients. They add amazing flavor and the fat you need to make it easy to stick to the keto life.

MEATLOAF

MAKES 4 SERVINGS

PREHEAT the oven to 400°F. Spray a loaf pan with cooking spray.

IN a bowl, mix together the ground beef, eggs, ketchup, pork rinds, onion, garlic, Italian seasoning, mustard, coconut aminos, and black pepper until thoroughly combined. I usually mix it with my (clean) hands, though a spoon works too.

TRANSFER the ground beef mixture to the prepared loaf pan and press evenly into the pan. Spread a little extra ketchup over the top of the meatloaf. Cover the pan with aluminum foil and bake for 1 hour, until cooked through.

WRAP any leftovers tightly in aluminum foil and refrigerate for 4 days, or freeze for up to 1 month.

NUTRITIONAL INFO (PER SERVING)
CALORIES 184, **FAT** 10.5 g, **PROTEIN** 8.3 g, **CARBS** 7.3 g, **FIBER** 15.7 g

VARIATIONS

MINI MEATLOAVES: If you have a smaller family or you're only cooking for yourself, you can make this in four mini loaf pans and freeze some to enjoy later. They will bake faster, so check for doneness after 40 minutes and watch carefully to avoid burning.

STUFFED MEATLOAF: Try stuffing cheese, spinach, olives, jalapeños, cream cheese, and/or soft-boiled eggs into the middle of the ground beef mixture (my favorite combo is cheddar, cream cheese, and jalapeños). You can also wrap the outside of the meatloaf in bacon before baking.

- 1½ pounds ground beef or ground pork (or a mixture of the two)
- 2 large eggs
- 5 tablespoons Homemade Sugar-Free Ketchup (page 237), plus extra to spread over the top
- ½ cup crushed pork rinds, ground flaxseed meal, or blanched almond flour
- ¼ cup chopped onion
- ½ teaspoon minced garlic
- 1 tablespoon dried Italian seasoning
- 1 tablespoon mustard powder
- 1 teaspoon coconut aminos (or soy sauce)
- ½ teaspoon ground black pepper

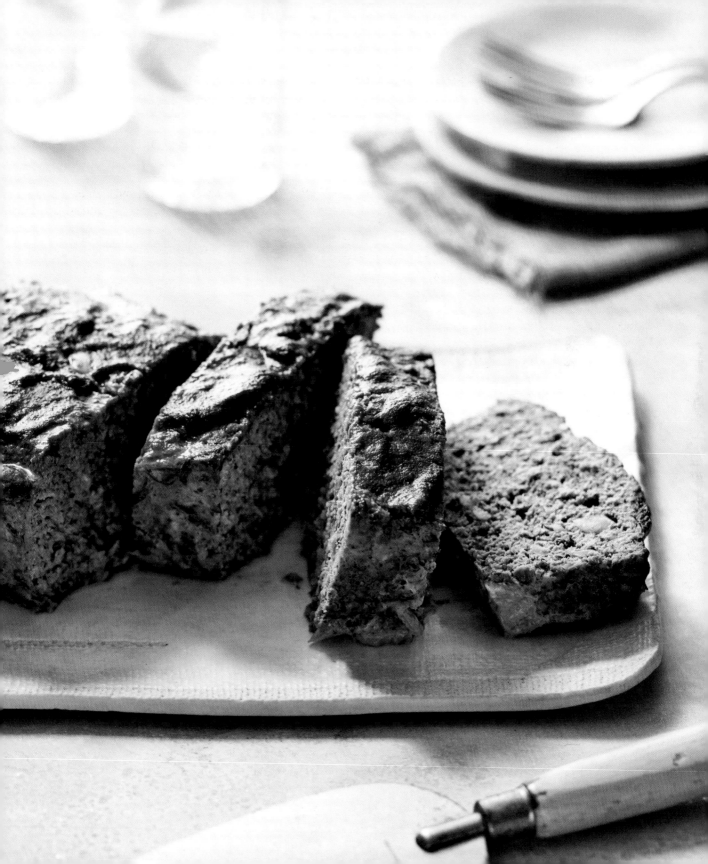

When you need a comforting and filling dinner, you can't do much better than shepherd's pie. It's meaty and bacony and cheesy in the best way possible, and it's still keto friendly. You can top it with ingredients like chopped fresh cilantro, sliced black olives, or crumbled cooked sugar-free nitrite-free bacon if you like.

SHEPHERD'S PIE

MAKES 8 SERVINGS

PREHEAT the oven to 375°F.

FOR THE FILLING

IN a large cast-iron pan over medium-high heat, heat the oil. Add the green and red peppers and the ground beef and cook, breaking up the beef with a wooden spoon, until the beef is browned. Add the bacon, black olives, eggs, chili powder, cumin, oregano, onion powder, salt, and pepper and mix thoroughly. Spread the mixture evenly in the pan and set aside.

FOR THE CAULIFLOWER

FILL a large pot with water and bring to a boil over high heat. Add the cauliflower and cook until tender, 5 to 7 minutes. Drain and roughly mash with a potato masher or an electric hand mixer. Add the cream and butter and continue mashing until smooth and creamy. Season with salt and pepper to taste.

SPREAD the cauliflower mash over the ground beef mixture. Sprinkle the shredded cheddar over the cauliflower. Bake for 20 to 25 minutes, until the cheese is melted and bubbly. Serve hot with optional toppings on the side.

NUTRITIONAL INFO (PER SERVING)
CALORIES 416, **FAT** 25.7 g, **PROTEIN** 31.9 g, **CARBS** 14.3 g, **FIBER** 2.2 g

BEEF FILLING

- 1 tablespoon extra-virgin olive oil
- ½ medium green bell pepper, seeded and diced
- ½ medium red bell pepper, seeded and diced
- 1½ pounds lean ground beef
- 6 slices sugar-free nitrite-free bacon, cooked and roughly chopped
- 2 ounces sliced black olives
- 3 large eggs, lightly beaten
- 1 tablespoon chili powder
- 1 teaspoon ground cumin
- 1 teaspoon dried oregano
- 1 teaspoon onion powder
- ¼ teaspoon salt
- ¼ teaspoon black pepper

MASHED CAULIFLOWER

- 1 head cauliflower, cut into florets
- ¼ cup heavy cream
- 3 tablespoons butter
- Salt and black pepper
- 2 cups shredded cheddar cheese

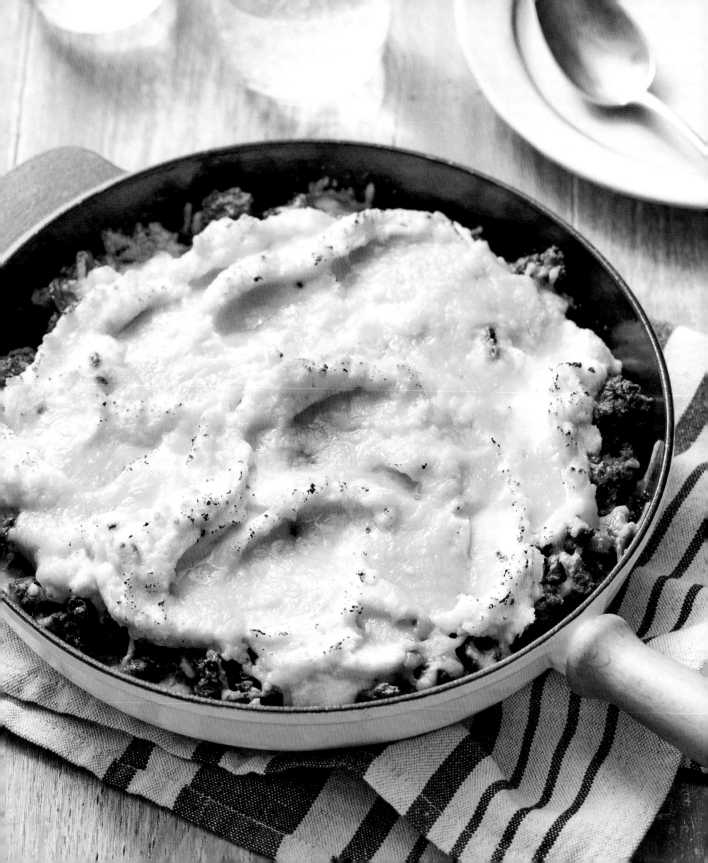

Cold, blustery days are made for bowls of hot chili. And this one is fabulous accompanied by Quick Keto Jalapeño Cheese Bread (page 30) or Low-Carb Biscuits (page 184). The secret ingredient is cocoa powder: A trick that has been passed down for generations, it adds a nice depth of flavor.

QUICK KETO CHILI

INSTANT POT OR PRESSURE COOKER METHOD

SET an Instant Pot or pressure cooker to sauté. Pour in the oil, add the onion, and cook, stirring, until translucent, 3 to 4 minutes. Add the ground beef and sausage and cook, breaking up the meat with a wooden spoon, until browned.

ADD the chili powder, cumin, cocoa powder, smoked paprika, garlic powder, oregano, salt, and pepper and stir until well combined. Add the broth, fire-roasted tomatoes, and Ro*Tel and stir. If you like a thicker chili, add the xanthan gum and stir to combine thoroughly.

SET the Instant Pot or pressure cooker on manual and cook on high pressure for 10 minutes. Use the quick release.

STOVETOP METHOD

IN a large pot over medium-high heat, warm the oil. Add the onion and cook, stirring, until translucent, 3 to 4 minutes. Add the ground beef and sausage and cook, breaking up the meat with a wooden spoon, until browned. Add the chili powder, cumin, cocoa powder, smoked paprika, garlic powder, oregano, salt, and pepper and stir until well combined. If you like a thicker chili, add the xanthan gum and stir to combine thoroughly. Add the bone broth, fire-roasted tomatoes, and Ro*Tel, stir to combine, and continue to cook until the chili begins to boil. Lower the heat to medium-low and simmer until the flavors meld, 10 to 12 minutes.

TO SERVE: Spoon the chili into bowls, top with shredded cheddar and sour cream, if using, and serve hot.

1 tablespoon extra-virgin olive oil

½ onion, diced

1 pound ground beef

1 pound bulk pork sausage

3 tablespoons chili powder

2 tablespoons ground cumin

1 tablespoon unsweetened cocoa powder

1 tablespoon smoked paprika

1 teaspoon garlic powder (or 2 teaspoons minced fresh garlic)

½ teaspoon dried oregano

1 teaspoon salt

1 teaspoon black pepper

2 cups Pressure Cooker Bone Broth (page 65) or store-bought bone broth

1 (15-ounce) can fire-roasted tomatoes

1 (10-ounce) can Ro*Tel mild diced tomatoes and green chilies

¼ teaspoon xanthan gum, optional, for extra thickness

OPTIONAL TOPPINGS

shredded cheddar cheese, sour cream

NUTRITIONAL INFO (PER SERVING)
CALORIES 200, **FAT** 7.8 g, **PROTEIN** 21.1 g, **CARBS** 12.4 g, **FIBER** 3.6 g

This might be the easiest pork chop recipe you will ever try. Pesto adds amazing flavors and oils to pork. Make my homemade pesto or purchase a tub at your local grocery store.

PARMESAN-CRUSTED PESTO PORK CHOPS

PREHEAT the oven to 350°F.

SEASON the pork chops with salt and pepper and place at least 1 inch apart in a large baking dish. Brush the pesto over the tops and sprinkle with the Parmesan.

BAKE for about 35 minutes, until an internal temperature of 145°F, or done to your liking.

NUTRITIONAL INFO (PER SERVING)
CALORIES 348, **FAT** 20.6 g, **PROTEIN** 38.4 g, **CARBS** 2.4 g, **FIBER** 0.3g

MAKES 4 SERVINGS

~~~

4 thin-cut boneless pork chops (about 4 ounces each)

1 teaspoon salt

1 teaspoon black pepper

4 teaspoons Basil Pesto (page 228)

¾ cup grated Parmesan cheese

Sometimes the simplest ingredients make the best meals. Pork tenderloin is one of my favorite cuts because it tastes great and is a wonderful base for lots of different flavors. Here we rub it with a few seasonings and roast it in the oven. Drizzle it with a simple butter pan sauce and dinner is served.

PERFECT PORK TENDERLOIN

PREHEAT the oven to 375°F.

FOR THE TENDERLOIN

MIX together the paprika, onion powder, garlic powder, salt, and pepper in a small bowl. Rub the tenderloin with the olive oil. Rub the seasoning mixture over the entire pork tenderloin.

HEAT a large ovenproof skillet over high heat. Place the tenderloin in the pan and sear for 1½ minutes without moving the pork. Turn and continue to sear until browned, 1½ minutes on each side.

TRANSFER the pan to the oven and roast for 10 to 15 minutes, until an instant-read thermometer inserted in the center reads 135°F to 145°F. Transfer the pork to a plate and let rest for about 5 minutes.

FOR THE PAN SAUCE

ADD the stock and butter to the pan and deglaze by scraping the browned bits off the bottom. Sprinkle in the xanthan gum and whisk until fully dissolved.

SLICE the tenderloin into ½-inch-thick pieces, drizzle the sauce over the top, and serve warm.

NUTRITIONAL INFO (PER SERVING)
CALORIES 386, **FAT** 19.8 g, **PROTEIN** 41.2 g, **CARBS** 12.1 g, **FIBER** 0.9 g

MAKES 4 SERVINGS

TENDERLOIN

2 teaspoons smoked paprika

½ teaspoon onion powder

½ teaspoon garlic powder

1 teaspoon salt

½ teaspoon black pepper

1½ to 2 pounds pork tenderloin, silver skin removed

2 tablespoons extra-virgin olive oil

PAN SAUCE

¼ cup Stovetop Chicken Stock (page 67) or store-bought chicken broth

2 tablespoons cold butter

½ teaspoon xanthan gum

PORK DONENESS TEMPERATURES
Medium-rare: 145°F
Medium: 150°F
Medium-well: 160°F

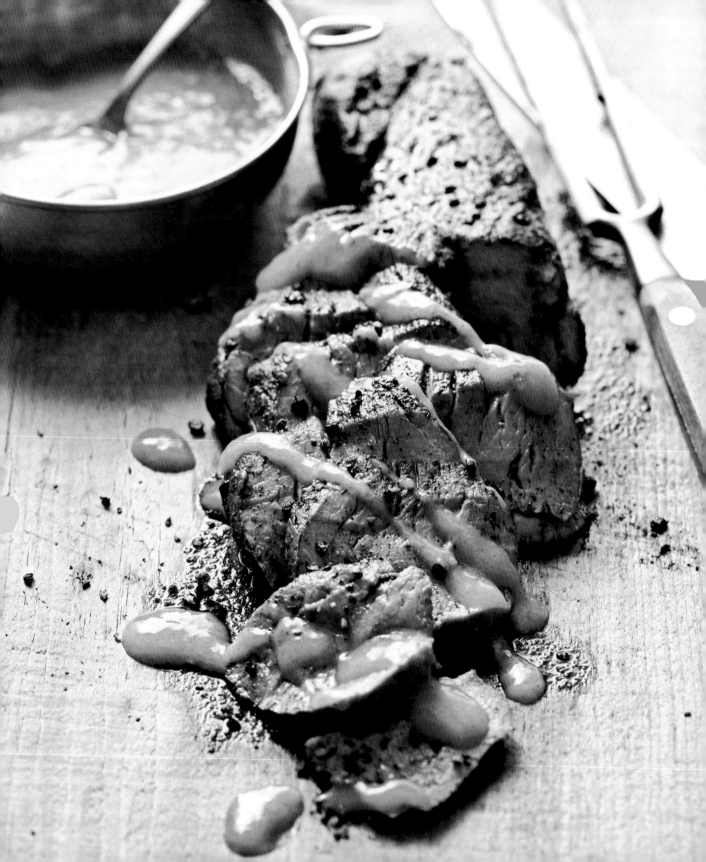

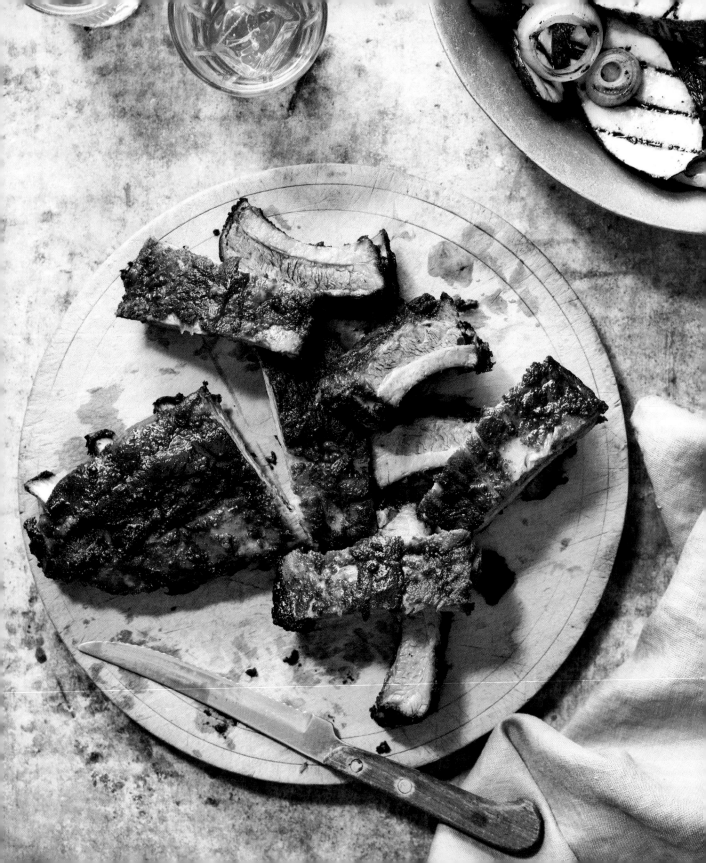

The ingredient that really makes this dish is mustard. It tenderizes the ribs without leaving any flavor. So if mustard isn't your favorite ingredient, please try it anyway—you'll never know it's there. Add a side of grilled vegetables and you'll have an amazing meal.

EASY OVEN-BAKED PORK RIBS

PREHEAT the oven to 250°F. Remove the membrane from the back side of the ribs using a small knife.

MIX together the sweetener, garlic powder, chili powder, paprika, onion powder, cayenne, salt, and white pepper in a small bowl. Rub the mixture onto the ribs on all sides. Spread the mustard all over the ribs.

WRAP the rack in foil and place on a baking sheet with the meat side down. Bake for 2 hours, until the meat is extremely tender.

NUTRITIONAL INFO (PER SERVING)
CALORIES 208, **FAT** 9.1 g, **PROTEIN** 26 g, **CARBS** 7.3 g, **FIBER** 2.2 g

**MAKES 2 SERVINGS
(½ RACK PER PERSON)**

~~~

1 rack baby back pork ribs (about 2 pounds)

1 tablespoon Sukrin Gold brown sugar sweetener

1 teaspoon garlic powder

1 teaspoon chili powder

1 teaspoon smoked paprika

½ teaspoon onion powder

½ teaspoon cayenne pepper

1 teaspoon salt

½ teaspoon white pepper

2 tablespoons mustard

Pork chops are one of my go-to cuts because they cook up quickly and go with so many flavors. The cheese here adds the fat you need to stay in ketosis and creates a really creamy sauce. Mushrooms add even more meaty flavor.

CREAMY ROSEMARY PORK CHOPS

SEASON the pork chops with salt and pepper.

IN a large skillet over medium heat, heat the olive oil. Add the pork chops and cook for about 2 minutes on each side. Transfer the chops to a plate and set aside.

ADD the mushrooms, onion, rosemary, and butter to the pan and cook, stirring, until the onion becomes slightly translucent, about 2 minutes. Add the stock and deglaze the pan by scraping the browned bits off the bottom. Add the mustard and mix with the stock until well combined. Add the cream, Parmesan, and cream cheese and mix until fully combined.

RETURN the pork chops to the pan, lower the heat, and simmer for about 10 minutes, until the sauce thickens.

NUTRITIONAL INFO (PER SERVING)
CALORIES 512, **FAT** 37.3 g, **PROTEIN** 39 g, **CARBS** 6.2 g, **FIBER** 1.3 g

MAKES 4 SERVINGS

~~~

- 4 thin-cut boneless pork chops (about 4 ounces each)
- 1 teaspoon salt
- 1 teaspoon black pepper
- 1 tablespoon extra-virgin olive oil
- 1 cup sliced cremini or button mushrooms
- 2 tablespoons chopped onion
- 2 tablespoons minced fresh rosemary
- 1 tablespoon butter
- 1/3 cup Stovetop Chicken Stock (page 67) or store-bought chicken broth
- 1 tablespoon Dijon mustard
- 1/2 cup heavy cream
- 1/2 cup grated Parmesan cheese
- 2 tablespoons cream cheese

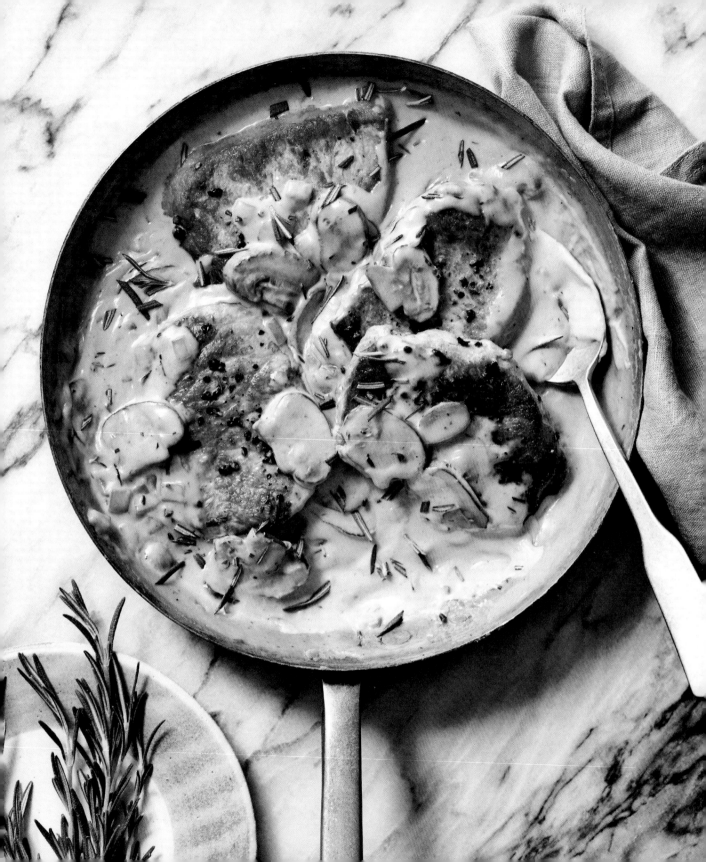

When dieting, many people crave something crispy that isn't a vegetable. These crispy chops will definitely satiate that craving with their crunchy coating of crushed pork rinds.

CRISPY PORK CHOPS

~~~

PREHEAT the oven to 350°F. Line a baking sheet with parchment paper or a silicone mat.

SEASON the pork chops on both sides with the salt and pepper.

IN a bowl, combine the pork rinds, egg white protein, parsley, sage, basil, oregano, and thyme. In another bowl, beat together the eggs and cream.

DIP each pork chop into the egg mixture and then dredge in the pork rind mixture. Lay the pork chops at least 1 inch apart on the prepared baking sheet. Bake for 23 to 25 minutes, until the internal temperature reaches 160°F.

NUTRITIONAL INFO (PER SERVING)
CALORIES 324, **FAT** 20.5 g, **PROTEIN** 31 g, **CARBS** 2 g, **FIBER** 0.2 g

6 center-cut (½-inch-thick)
    pork chops
    (about 4 ounces each)

1 teaspoon salt

½ teaspoon black pepper

3 ounces pork rinds, crushed

1 tablespoon egg white
    protein or unflavored whey
    protein isolate

1 teaspoon chopped fresh
    parsley

1 teaspoon dried sage

½ teaspoon dried basil

½ teaspoon dried oregano

½ teaspoon dried thyme

2 large eggs

2 tablespoons heavy cream

It's always good to have a reliable casserole you can throw together and bring to a potluck or a party so you can be sure there will be something for you to eat. This is it. You will never feel left out when you make this. And everyone else will love it too.

PORK SAUSAGE CASSEROLE

PREHEAT the oven to 350°F. Spray a 9- by 13-inch baking dish with cooking spray.

IN a large skillet over medium heat, melt the butter. Add the mushrooms, celery, and onion and cook, stirring, until the onion is translucent, 2 to 3 minutes. Add the sausage and continue to cook, breaking up the sausage with a wooden spoon, until browned, 4 to 5 minutes.

ADD the cauliflower rice and cook until the cauliflower is slightly tender, another 3 to 4 minutes. Remove the skillet from the heat and set aside to cool for 5 minutes.

IN a large bowl, mix together the beaten eggs, cream, parsley, thyme, sage, rosemary, garlic powder, salt, and pepper. Add the sausage mixture to the egg mixture and mix well. Transfer the mixture to the prepared baking dish. If using, sprinkle the cheddar cheese over the sausage mixture. Bake for 20 to 25 minutes, until a knife comes out clean when inserted into the center of the casserole.

MAKES 6 SERVINGS

2 tablespoons butter

8 ounces cremini mushrooms, sliced

2 stalks celery, minced

1 small onion, minced

1 pound bulk pork sausage

1 cup riced cauliflower

4 large eggs, beaten

½ cup heavy cream

1 teaspoon chopped fresh parsley

1 teaspoon dried thyme

1 teaspoon dried sage

1 teaspoon dried rosemary

1 teaspoon garlic powder

1 teaspoon salt

½ teaspoon black pepper

½ cup shredded cheddar cheese, optional

NUTRITIONAL INFO (PER SERVING)
CALORIES 229, **FAT** 18.4 g, **PROTEIN** 9.7 g, **CARBS** 7.7 g, **FIBER** 1.7 g

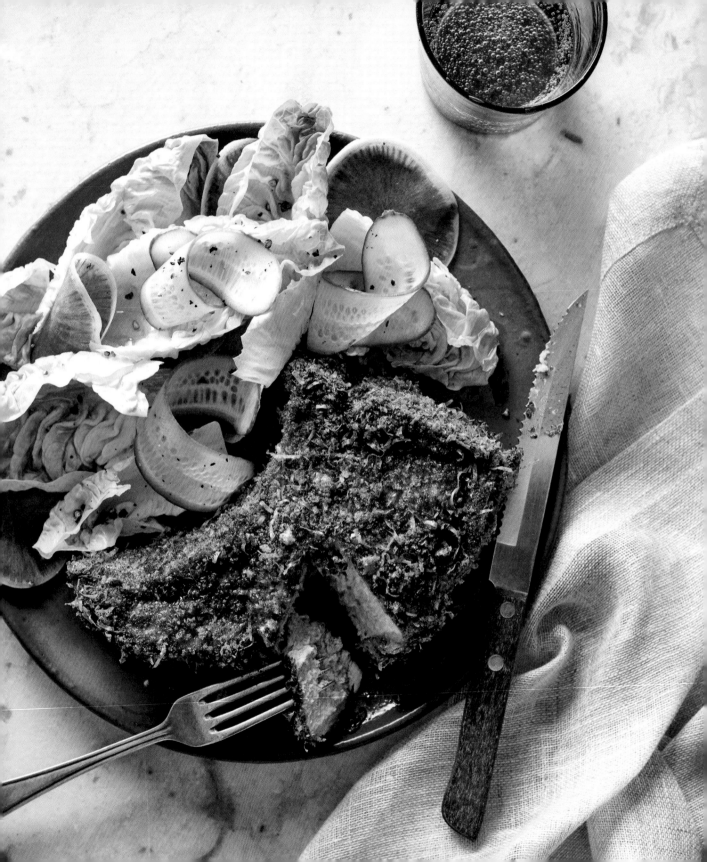

For the crispiest results, I like to use the air fryer for this recipe. But if you don't have one, I've included a stovetop method because I don't want anyone to miss making these really yummy pork chops. Bone-in chops will also work. Serve with the Creamy Cucumber Salad (page 56) or a simple side salad.

AIR-FRYER PARMESAN-CRUSTED PORK CHOPS

MAKES 4 SERVINGS

~~~

6 center-cut (½-inch-thick) boneless pork chops (about 4 ounces each)

½ teaspoon salt

¼ teaspoon black pepper

1 cup crushed pork rinds

3 tablespoons grated Parmesan cheese

1 teaspoon smoked paprika

½ teaspoon onion powder

¼ teaspoon chili powder

2 large eggs

1 tablespoon olive oil (if cooking on the stovetop)

SEASON both sides of the pork chops with the salt and pepper. In a medium bowl, combine the pork rind crumbs, Parmesan, paprika, onion powder, and chili powder. In another medium bowl, beat the eggs. Dip each pork chop into the egg mixture and then immediately dredge in the pork rind mixture, making sure to cover them completely with the crumbs.

AIR FRYER METHOD

PREHEAT the air fryer to 400°F. Place three pork chops in the air fryer basket and cook for 12 to 15 minutes, until crispy and the internal temperature reaches 160°F. Repeat to cook the remaining chops.

STOVETOP METHOD

PLACE a large cast-iron skillet over medium-high heat. Add the olive oil and heat until almost smoking. Add the pork chops and cook for 2 to 3 minutes, turn, and cook for another 1 to 2 minutes, until browned and cooked through.

NUTRITIONAL INFO (PER SERVING)
CALORIES 319, **FAT** 11.5 g, **PROTEIN** 19.3 g, **CARBS** 1.1 g, **FIBER** 0.4 g

Egg rolls are one of the most popular Chinese appetizers, but when you're on a keto diet the wrappers are a no-no. Here, they're deconstructed so you get all the flavors of egg rolls while still maintaining ketosis. It makes a great light lunch.

EGG ROLL IN A BOWL

IN a small skillet over medium-low heat, heat the olive oil. Add the beaten eggs and cook, stirring, until scrambled. Set aside.

IN a large skillet over medium-high heat, heat the sesame oil and add the ground pork, salt, and pepper. Cook, breaking up the pork with a wooden spoon, until browned, 6 to 7 minutes. Add ½ cup of the green onions, the ginger, and garlic. Lower the heat to medium and continue to cook, stirring, for 3 minutes.

CAREFULLY add the coleslaw mixture and cook, stirring, until the slaw is tender, about 10 minutes. Pour in the coconut aminos, add the scrambled eggs, and cook, stirring, until cooked through, 1 minute longer. Taste and season with additional salt and pepper if needed.

TRANSFER to a serving bowl and top with the remaining ½ cup chopped green onions and a sprinkle of sesame seeds.

LEFTOVERS can be refrigerated, covered, for up to 2 days.

MAKES 8 SERVINGS

〜〜〜

1 teaspoon extra-virgin olive oil

2 large eggs, lightly beaten

1 teaspoon sesame oil

1 pound ground pork

1½ teaspoons salt

1 teaspoon black pepper

1 cup chopped green onions

2 tablespoons grated fresh ginger

1 tablespoon minced garlic

16 ounces tricolor coleslaw mixture

¼ cup coconut aminos or soy sauce

Sesame seeds, for garnish

NUTRITIONAL INFO (PER SERVING)
CALORIES 576, **FAT** 41.4 g, **PROTEIN** 39.2 g, **CARBS** 10.8 g, **FIBER** 3.4 g

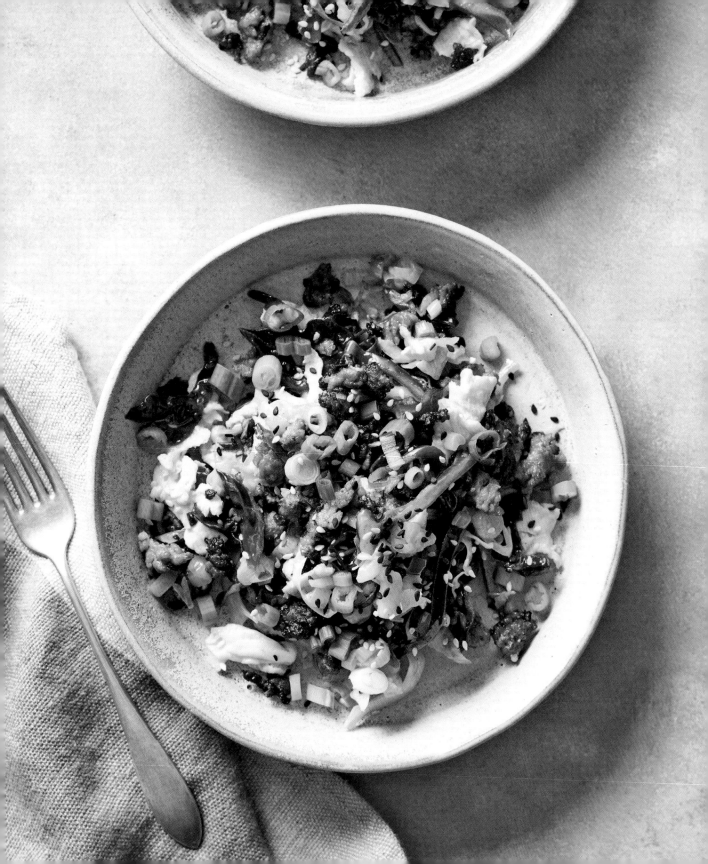

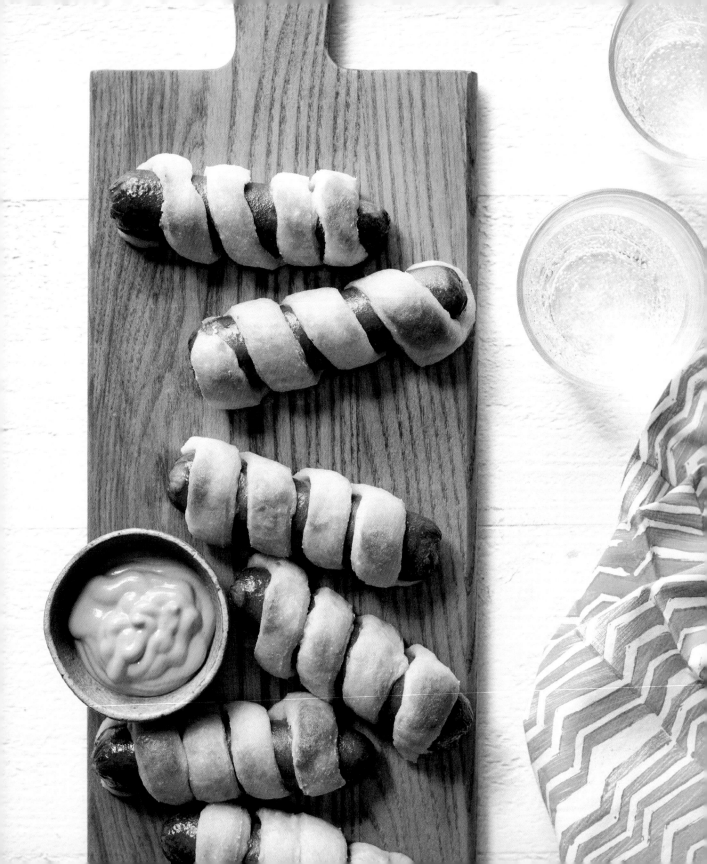

Everyone loves pigs in a blanket, and I was so glad to figure out how to make the "blanket" without traditional flour. My family loves these, so I think I was successful.

LOW-CARB PIGS IN A BLANKET

PREHEAT the oven to 350°F. Line a baking sheet with parchment paper or a silicone mat.

IN a microwave-safe bowl, mix together the mozzarella, almond flour, and cream cheese and heat in the microwave oven for 1 minute. Add the egg and mix it into the other ingredients until they come together into a dough. Let the dough cool for 2 to 3 minutes.

PLACE a sheet of parchment paper on the counter. Place the dough on the parchment and place another sheet the same size on top. Using a rolling pin, roll the dough into a rectangle about 9 by 13 inches and ¼ inch thick. With a pizza cutter, cut the dough lengthwise into 1-inch strips. (If there is any leftover dough, roll it into a ball and bake it as a biscuit along with the pigs in a blanket.)

WRAP one strip of dough around one of the hot dogs in a spiral. Sometimes the dough can become sticky and hard to handle. I usually keep a dish towel nearby and dry my hands after wrapping each hot dog to minimize this.

REPEAT to wrap all the hot dogs, placing each pig in a blanket on the prepared baking sheet. Bake for 20 minutes, until the crust becomes golden brown.

SERVE with mustard, ketchup, or whatever condiments you like on the side.

NUTRITIONAL INFO (PER SERVING)
CALORIES 245, **FAT** 14.4 g, **PROTEIN** 14.6 g, **CARBS** 3.9 g, **FIBER** 1.1 g

MAKES 8 SERVINGS

~~~

1¾ cups shredded part-skim low-moisture mozzarella cheese

¾ cup blanched almond flour

2 tablespoons cream cheese

1 large egg

8 nitrate-free hot dogs

OPTIONAL ACCOMPANIMENTS
mustard, ketchup

VARIATION
Make small, appetizer-sized pigs in a blanket using cocktail hot dogs or sausages. Cut the dough into shorter lengths and wrap around each small hot dog. Bake as instructed in the recipe, checking at 15 minutes to make sure they don't burn.

You'll find yourself making this dough frequently once you realize all the different ingredients you can use to stuff it. Take your pick from the three fillings below, or create your own. Don't forget to use parchment or a silicone mat when rolling out the dough or it will stick to the counter and be a mess to clean up.

POCKET DOUGH DINNER—THREE WAYS

PREHEAT the oven to 350°F. Have a silicone mat ready or a large piece of parchment paper. Line a baking sheet with parchment paper.

FOR THE BEEF FILLING
IN a small skillet over medium-high heat, heat the oil. Add the ground beef and cook, breaking it up with a wooden spoon, until browned. Let cool. Add the mozzarella and jalapeño and mix together until combined. Set aside.

FOR THE ITALIAN FILLING
IN a small skillet over medium-high heat, heat the oil. Add the ground beef and cook, breaking it up with a wooden spoon, until browned. Add the marinara, oregano, basil, salt, and pepper and mix together until combined. Set aside.

FOR THE PEPPERONI PIZZA FILLING
IN a small skillet over medium-high heat, cook the sausage, breaking it up with a wooden spoon, until browned. Add the pepperoni, cheddar, and marinara and mix until combined. Set aside.

FOR THE DOUGH
MIX together the almond flour, coconut flour, baking powder, garlic powder, onion powder, and salt in a bowl.

MAKES 8 SERVINGS

~~~

CHEESY BEEF FILLING

2 tablespoons extra-virgin olive oil

1 pound ground beef

½ cup shredded part-skim low-moisture mozzarella cheese

2 tablespoons chopped seeded fresh jalapeño pepper

ITALIAN FILLING

2 tablespoons extra-virgin olive oil

1 pound ground beef

½ cup Homemade Marinara Sauce (page 236)

1 teaspoon dried oregano

1 teaspoon dried basil

½ teaspoon salt

¼ teaspoon black pepper

PEPPERONI PIZZA FILLING

8 ounces bulk pork sausage

8 ounces pepperoni, chopped

½ cup shredded cheddar cheese

½ cup Homemade Marinara Sauce (page 236)

POCKET DOUGH

½ cup blanched almond flour

¼ cup coconut flour

1½ teaspoons baking powder

½ teaspoon garlic powder

½ teaspoon onion powder

½ teaspoon salt

1¾ cups shredded part-skim low-moisture mozzarella cheese

5 tablespoons butter

1 large egg

IN a medium saucepan over low heat, melt the mozzarella. Remove from the heat, add the butter and egg, and mix together thoroughly. Add the flour mixture to the saucepan and mix together. It may take a while for the dough to come together. The dough should be warm at this point but not hot.

TRANSFER the dough to the silicone mat or parchment paper. (I prefer the silicone mat because it sticks to the counter and doesn't move around when you are rolling out the dough.) Divide the dough in half.

USING a rolling pin, gently roll out one warm dough portion into a 9- by 13-inch rectangle and set aside. Repeat with the second piece of dough. If the dough becomes sticky and hard to roll, sprinkle with a little bit of coconut flour.

TO fill the pocket dough, spoon half of whichever filling you made into the center of one rectangle of dough. Fold the dough over into a rectangle and seal the edges by pressing the dough with your fingers or using the tines of a fork. With a sharp knife, cut two or three vents in the top of the dough. Repeat with the remaining filling and dough.

PLACE the two filled pocket doughs on the prepared baking sheet and bake for 20 minutes, until the tops are browned.

SERVE hot. Place any leftovers in zip-top plastic bags and store in the refrigerator for up to 4 days. To reheat, simply place in the microwave for about 30 seconds to 1 minute until warm.

NUTRITIONAL INFO (PER SERVING) FOR DOUGH ONLY
CALORIES 178, **FAT** 15.4 g, **PROTEIN** 7.6 g, **CARBS** 6 g, **FIBER** 2.1 g

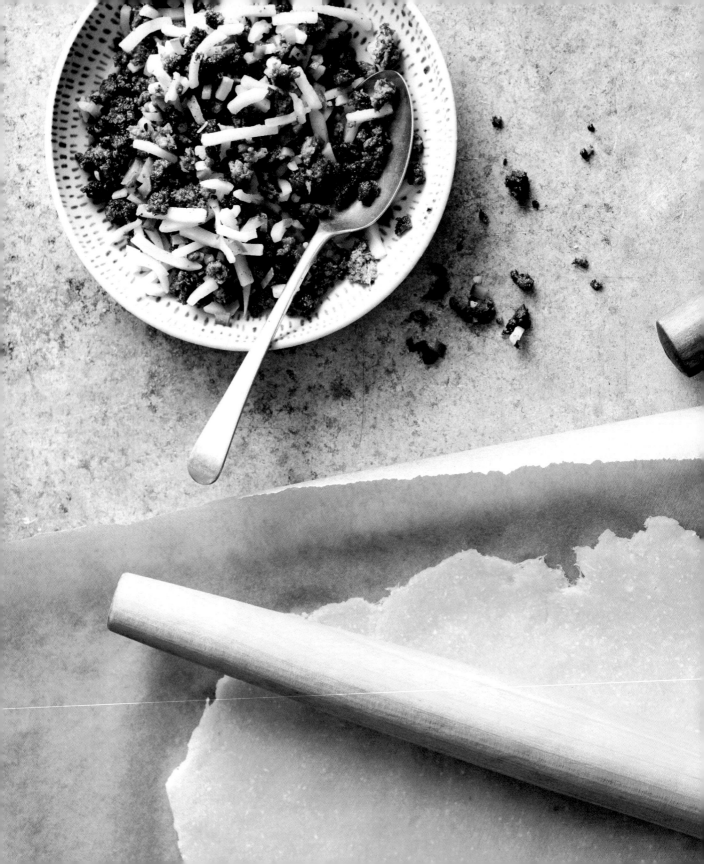

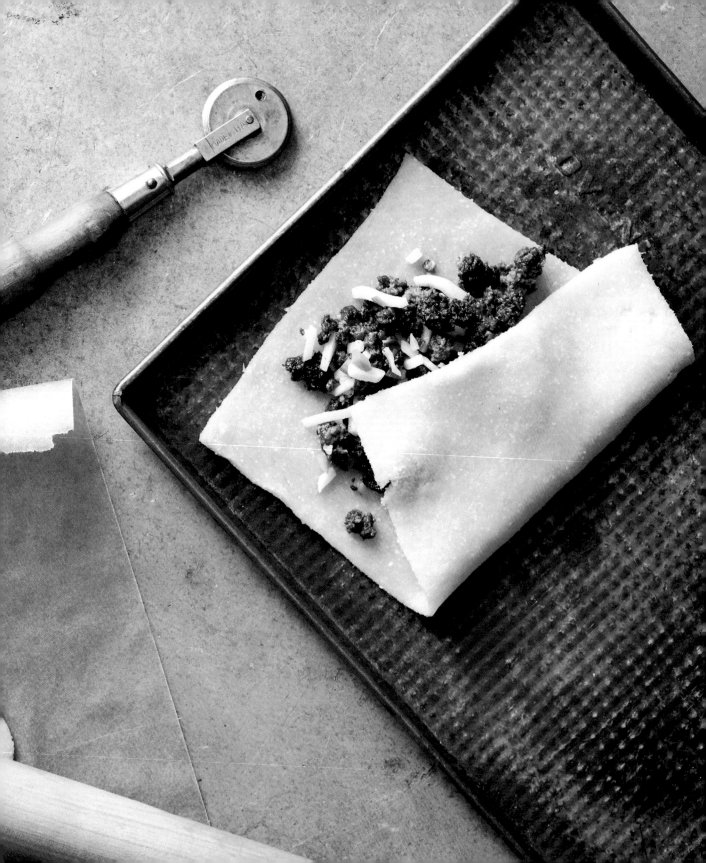

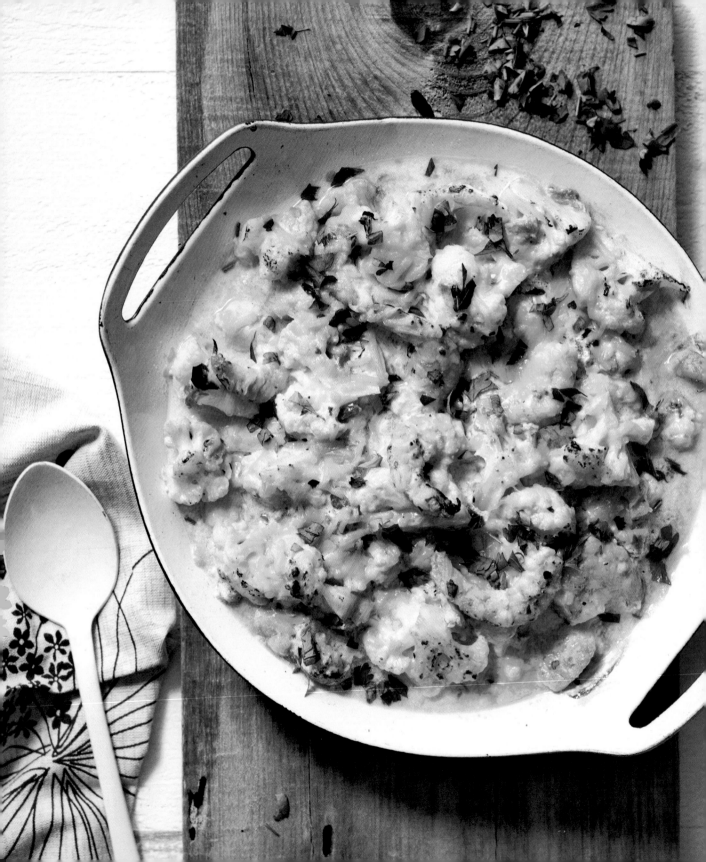

Try making this for an easy weeknight meal. It comes together very quickly and requires very little hands-on time.

EASY SHRIMP CASSEROLE

PREHEAT the oven to 350°F. Have a 9- by 13-inch baking dish ready.

PLACE the frozen cauliflower in a microwave-safe bowl and heat in the microwave oven for about 5 minutes, until tender.

IN a large bowl, mix together the cauliflower, Ro*tel, ½ cup of the cheddar, the cream cheese, sour cream, hot sauce, lemon zest and juice, garlic, salt, pepper, and red pepper flakes until fully combined. Add the shrimp and mix together.

POUR the mixture into the baking dish and top with the remaining ½ cup shredded cheddar. Bake for 35 to 40 minutes, until bubbly and cooked through.

SPRINKLE with the parsley and serve.

NUTRITIONAL INFO (PER SERVING)
CALORIES 259, **FAT** 14.9 g, **PROTEIN** 23.5 g, **CARBS** 9.7 g, **FIBER** 2 g

MAKES 6 SERVINGS

~~~~

- 1 (16-ounce) bag frozen cauliflower florets
- 1 (10-ounce) can Ro*tel mild diced tomatoes and green chilies, drained
- 1 cup shredded cheddar cheese
- 4 ounces cream cheese, softened
- ¼ cup sour cream
- 3 tablespoons Frank's RedHot hot sauce
- 1 teaspoon grated lemon zest
- 2 tablespoons lemon juice
- 1 tablespoon minced garlic
- ½ teaspoon salt
- ½ teaspoon black pepper
- ¼ teaspoon red pepper flakes
- 1 pound cooked frozen shrimp, thawed
- 2 tablespoons minced fresh parsley

This is a recipe that comes together very quickly if you have a spiralizer, but a mandoline will still do the job. The scampi is actually quite pretty with its bright cherry tomatoes and green zucchini.

SKILLET SHRIMP SCAMPI WITH ZOODLES

USING a spiralizer, cut the zucchini into zoodles. Alternatively, you can cut the zucchini into thin strips with a mandoline or vegetable peeler. Set aside.

IN a large skillet over medium-high heat, melt the butter. Add the broth, 1 tablespoon of the olive oil, the garlic, salt, and pepper and simmer, stirring, until heated through, 2 to 3 minutes. Add the shrimp and cook, stirring, until they turn pink, 2 to 3 minutes. Transfer the shrimp and sauce to a bowl and set aside.

ADD the remaining 1 tablespoon oil to the skillet, add the zoodles, and cook over medium-high heat, stirring, just until they become tender, 3 to 5 minutes. Return the shrimp mixture to the skillet with the zoodles and cook, stirring, for another minute, until heated through.

TRANSFER to a serving bowl, sprinkle with the lemon juice, add cherry tomatoes, if using, and serve.

NUTRITIONAL INFO (PER SERVING)
CALORIES 212, **FAT** 9.4 g, **PROTEIN** 30.9 g, **CARBS** 2 g, **FIBER** 0.4 g

MAKES 6 SERVINGS

~~~

3 medium zucchini

2 tablespoons butter

½ cup store-bought vegetable broth (or broth from Old-Fashioned Vegetable Soup, page 68)

2 tablespoons extra-virgin olive oil

2 teaspoons minced garlic

½ teaspoon salt

¼ teaspoon black pepper

2 pounds large shrimp, peeled and deveined

1 tablespoon lemon juice

Halved cherry tomatoes, optional

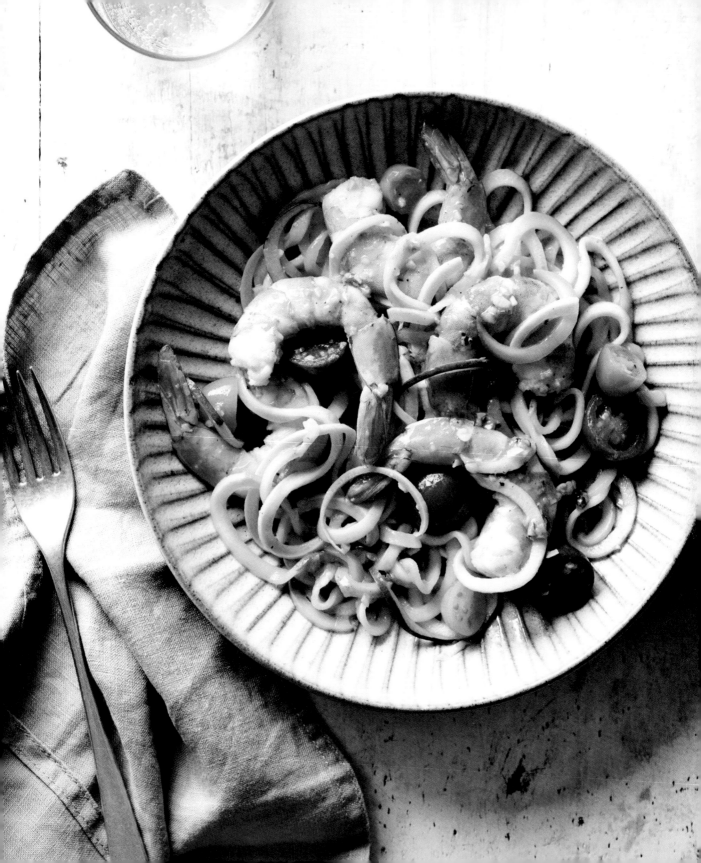

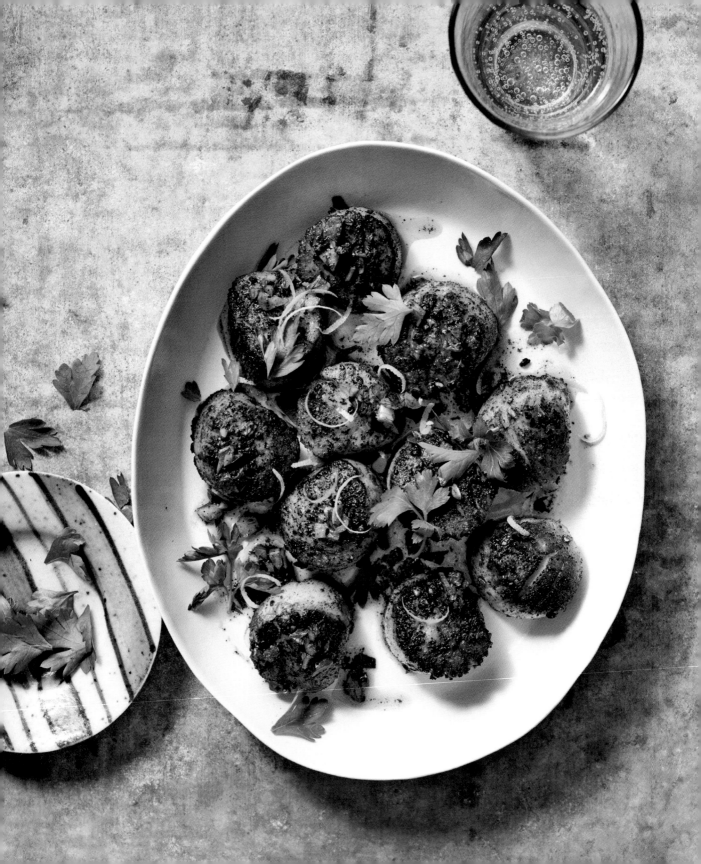

You can make this dish with shrimp instead of scallops, but don't increase the heat when you add them to the pan. This also tastes great with tilapia or cod. Serve with cauliflower rice or a side salad.

GARLIC SCALLOPS

SEASON the scallops with the salt, pepper, and paprika.

IN a skillet over medium heat, warm the olive oil. Add the garlic and cook, stirring, for about 1 minute. Increase the heat to medium-high, add the scallops, and cook until browned, 2 to 3 minutes on each side. Stir in the butter, lemon juice, and half the parsley.

TRANSFER the scallops to a serving platter and drizzle with the sauce from the pan. Sprinkle the grated lemon zest and remaining parsley over the top right before serving.

NOTE: *Don't have smoked paprika? Add a pinch of cumin to regular paprika and you will get the same smoky flavor.*

NUTRITIONAL INFO (PER SERVING)
CALORIES 193, **FAT** 18.8 g, **PROTEIN** 1.9 g, **CARBS** 6.7 g, **FIBER** 1.6 g

MAKES 4 SERVINGS

~~~

- 1 pound large scallops
- 1 teaspoon salt
- ½ teaspoon black pepper
- ¼ teaspoon smoked paprika (see Note)
- 2 tablespoons extra-virgin olive oil
- 3 tablespoons minced garlic
- 4 tablespoons salted butter
- 2 tablespoons lemon juice
- ¼ cup chopped fresh parsley
- 1 teaspoon grated lemon zest

Bacon and fish are great flavor partners and this recipe is no exception. It's a complete weeknight meal that will be ready in about 30 minutes.

BACON-WRAPPED COD WITH LEMON-CAPER SPINACH

PAT the cod fillets dry with a paper towel and sprinkle with the salt and pepper. Wrap each fillet with 1 slice of bacon.

MELT the butter in a large skillet over medium heat. Add the bacon-wrapped fillets and cook until the fish flakes easily with a fork, 4 to 5 minutes on each side. Transfer the fillets to a plate.

RETURN the skillet to the heat. Add the garlic and cook, stirring, until fragrant, about 30 seconds. Add the spinach, capers, and lemon juice and cook, stirring occasionally, until the spinach wilts, about 2 minutes.

TRANSFER the spinach to a serving plate and top with the cod fillets. Sprinkle with the lemon zest and serve.

NUTRITIONAL INFO (PER SERVING)
CALORIES 315, **FAT** 11.6 g, **PROTEIN** 24.5 g, **CARBS** 5.9 g, **FIBER** 2 g

MAKES 2 SERVINGS

~~~~

4 cod fillets (8 ounces each)

½ teaspoon salt

¼ teaspoon black pepper

4 slices sugar-free nitrite-free thin-cut bacon

1 tablespoon butter

½ teaspoon minced garlic

4 cups fresh spinach

2 tablespoons drained capers

1 teaspoon lemon juice

½ teaspoon grated lemon zest

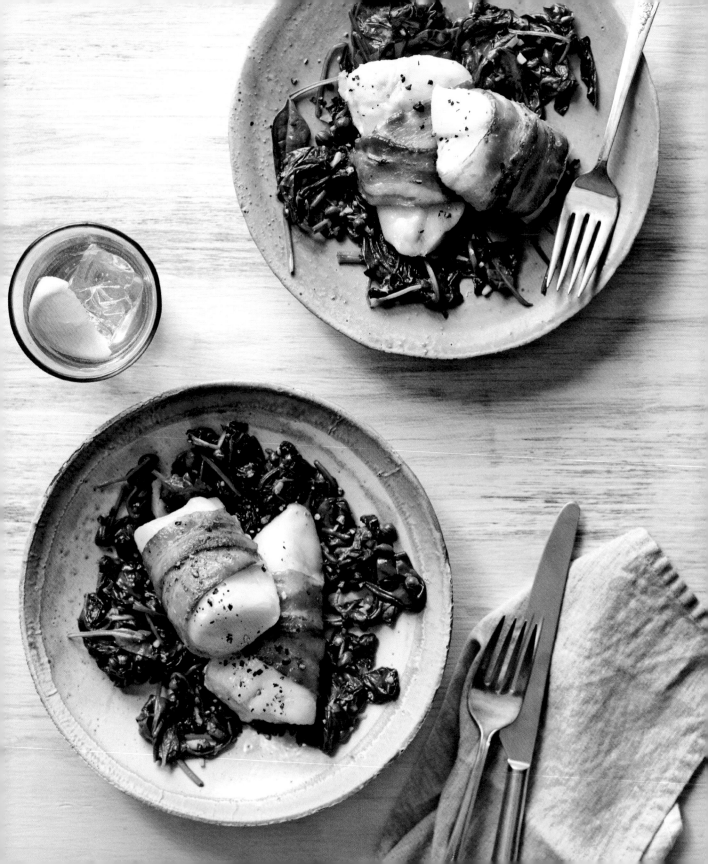

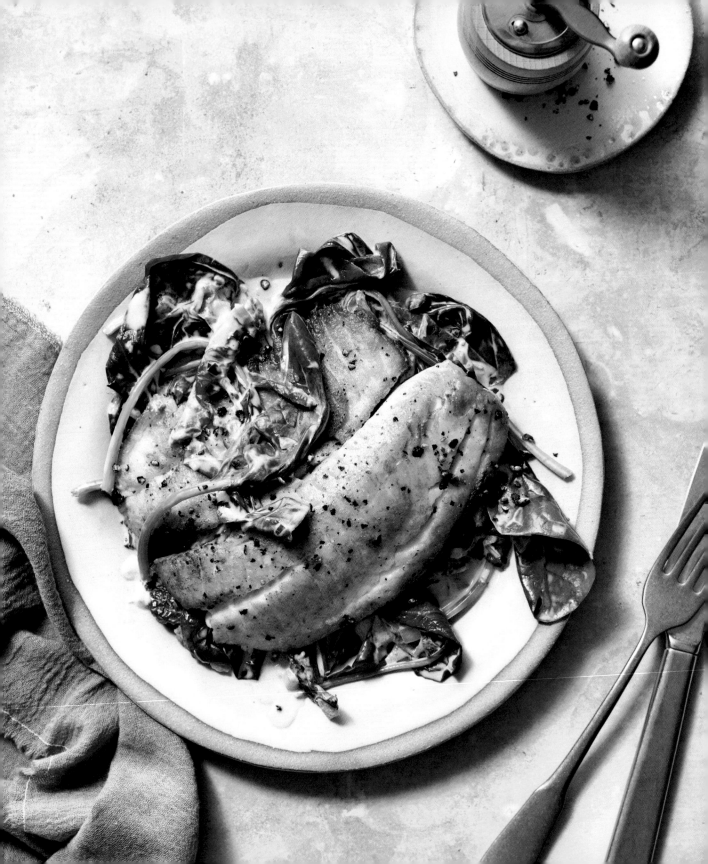

In this Italian classic, I use tilapia instead of the more traditional chicken because it goes perfectly with sun-dried tomatoes and spinach. Any firm white fish will work for this dish, including cod or halibut. It has a lovely creamy sauce, with sun-dried tomatoes contributing little explosions of flavor.

TUSCAN-STYLE TILAPIA

SEASON the tilapia fillets on both sides with the salt and pepper.

IN a large skillet, heat the olive oil over medium heat. Add the tilapia and cook until it flakes easily with a fork, 3 to 4 minutes on each side. Transfer the fillets to a plate and keep warm.

RETURN the pan to the heat. Add the onion and garlic and cook, stirring, until the onion is translucent, about 3 minutes. Add the broth and cook, stirring, for about 3 minutes. Add the cream, sun-dried tomatoes, parsley, and cream cheese and cook, stirring, for 5 to 6 minutes. Add the spinach and cook, stirring occasionally, until the spinach wilts, about 3 minutes.

TRANSFER to a serving plate, top with the tilapia fillets, sprinkle with parsley, and serve.

NUTRITIONAL INFO (PER SERVING)
CALORIES 425, **FAT** 30.8 g, **PROTEIN** 28.5 g, **CARBS** 12.3 g, **FIBER** 3 g

MAKES 4 SERVINGS

~~~

4 or 5 tilapia fillets (6 ounces each)

1 teaspoon salt

¼ teaspoon black pepper

2 tablespoons extra-virgin olive oil

1 yellow onion, diced

1 tablespoon minced garlic

½ cup vegetable broth (or broth from Old-Fashioned Vegetable Soup, page 68) or seafood broth

¾ cup heavy cream

½ cup sliced sun-dried tomatoes

2 tablespoons minced fresh parsley, plus more for garnish

1 tablespoon cream cheese, at room temperature

4 cups fresh spinach

Pico de gallo, a mixture of chopped tomato, onion, and a little jalapeño, is available at your grocery store, but you can make it yourself too. These savory cakes get a little kick from the pico de gallo, and they pair very well with a simple side salad for a terrific light lunch.

TUNA CAKES

MAKES 6 SERVINGS

~~~~

2 (5-ounce) cans tuna in water, drained

2 large eggs

½ cup shredded Colby Jack cheese

4 ounces pork rinds, crushed into crumbs

2 tablespoons pico de gallo, plus more for serving

½ cup coconut oil

Chopped fresh cilantro, for garnish

IN a bowl, mix together the tuna, eggs, shredded cheese, crushed pork rinds, and pico de gallo and mix until fully combined. Divide the mixture into 6 round patties.

IN a large skillet, melt the coconut oil over medium-high heat. Add the tuna cakes and cook until golden brown, 2 to 3 minutes on each side.

SPRINKLE the cakes with cilantro and serve with additional pico de gallo on the side.

NUTRITIONAL INFO (PER SERVING)
CALORIES 473, **FAT** 44 g, **PROTEIN** 17.2 g, **CARBS** 0.9 g, **FIBER** 0 g

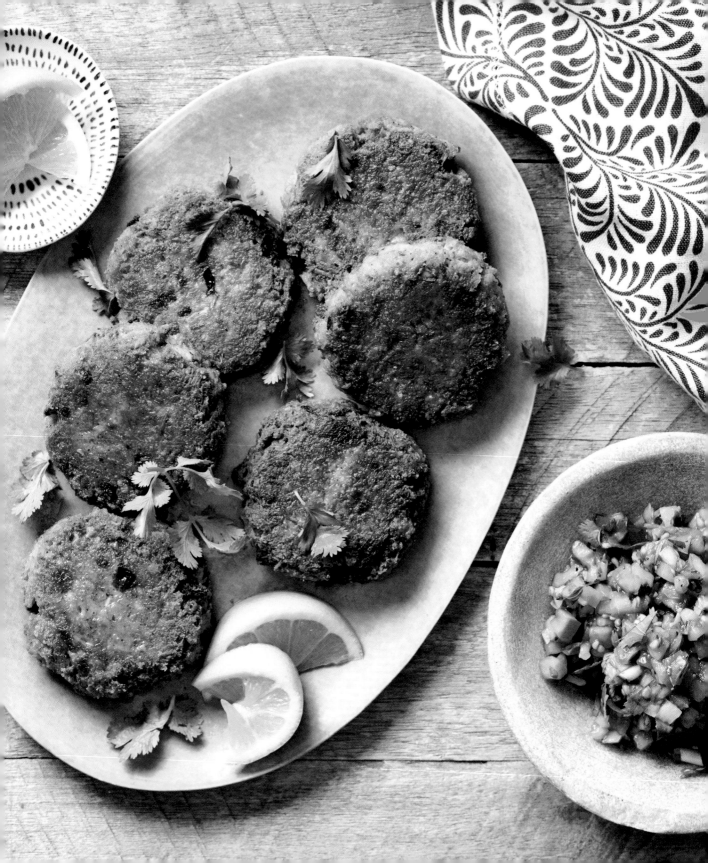

Make this casserole when you need a super-fast dinner because you forgot to defrost anything beforehand. (And haven't we all done that?) Sriracha is an Asian hot sauce that I like very much, but feel free to use the hot sauce of your choice.

BROCCOLI TUNA CASSEROLE

PREHEAT the oven to 350°F. Have a 9- by 13-inch baking dish ready.

COOK the broccoli florets in the microwave as instructed on the package. Layer the broccoli in the baking dish and set aside.

IN a bowl, mix together the tuna, mayo, ketchup, mustard, and sriracha until well blended. Spread the mixture over the top of the broccoli florets in the baking dish. Top with the shredded cheese. Bake for 25 to 30 minutes, until the casserole is bubbly and the cheese starts to brown.

NUTRITIONAL INFO (PER SERVING)
CALORIES 476, **FAT** 39.3 g, **PROTEIN** 25.9 g, **CARBS** 5 g, **FIBER** 2.1 g

MAKES 6 SERVINGS

~~~

1 (12-ounce) bag frozen broccoli florets

3 (5-ounce) cans tuna in water, drained

1 cup Homemade Mayo (page 229)

2 tablespoons Homemade Sugar-Free Ketchup (page 237)

2 tablespoons yellow mustard

2 teaspoons sriracha

1 cup shredded Colby Jack cheese

This recipe is perfect for large groups of people because it can easily be doubled. Don't use imitation crab—use real, fresh crabmeat that you'll find in your local grocery store's seafood section.

CRABMEAT CASSEROLE

PREHEAT the oven to 350°F. Spray a 9- by 9-inch baking dish with cooking spray.

MELT the butter in a saucepan over medium-high heat. Add the onion and cook, stirring, until translucent, 2 to 3 minutes.

IN a bowl, beat the egg whites until they form soft peaks, 5 to 6 minutes. Set aside.

IN another bowl, mix together the cooked onion, egg yolks, crabmeat, mustard, hot sauce, Worcestershire sauce, salt, and pepper. Fold the beaten egg whites into the crab mixture and transfer the mixture to the prepared baking dish. Sprinkle the Parmesan and cheddar over the top.

BAKE for 25 minutes, until puffy and golden brown. Let cool for 5 minutes, then cut into squares and serve.

NUTRITIONAL INFO (PER SERVING)
CALORIES 191, **FAT** 9.8 g, **PROTEIN** 22.3 g, **CARBS** 2.2 g, **FIBER** 0.4 g

MAKES 6 SERVINGS

1 teaspoon butter

¼ cup chopped onion

5 large eggs, separated

1 pound fresh crabmeat

2 tablespoons Dijon mustard

2 tablespoons Frank's RedHot hot sauce

1 teaspoon Worcestershire sauce

1 teaspoon salt

½ teaspoon black pepper

2 tablespoons grated Parmesan cheese

½ cup shredded cheddar cheese

5

SIDE DISHES

Look for nitrite-free sugar-free bacon. I like thinly sliced bacon for this recipe, but thick-cut bacon works well too. But you might need to roast the asparagus a few minutes longer to make sure the bacon gets crisp.

BACON-WRAPPED ASPARAGUS

PREHEAT the oven to 400°F. Line a baking sheet with parchment paper or a silicone mat.

TRIM the asparagus by breaking off the ends. Rinse and pat dry. Wrap a slice of bacon in a spiral around each stalk of asparagus. (A full slice of bacon will work for larger stalks of asparagus; cut the bacon strips in half for shorter stalks.) Arrange the asparagus on the prepared baking sheet, making sure they don't touch.

IN a small saucepan over medium heat, melt the butter with the syrup, if using, and coconut aminos until a bit thick and bubbly. Baste the asparagus with the syrup mixture.

BAKE for about 20 minutes, until the bacon becomes brown and crispy to your liking.

MAKES 4 SERVINGS

~~~

1 pound large asparagus (12 to 16 stalks)

6 to 16 slices thin-cut sugar-free nitrite-free bacon

8 tablespoons butter

1 tablespoon Homemade Maple Syrup (page 241) or other sugar-free syrup, optional

1 teaspoon coconut aminos

NUTRITIONAL INFO (PER SERVING)
CALORIES 143, **FAT** 12.3 g, **PROTEIN** 3.6 g, **CARBS** 4.8 g, **FIBER** 5.1 g

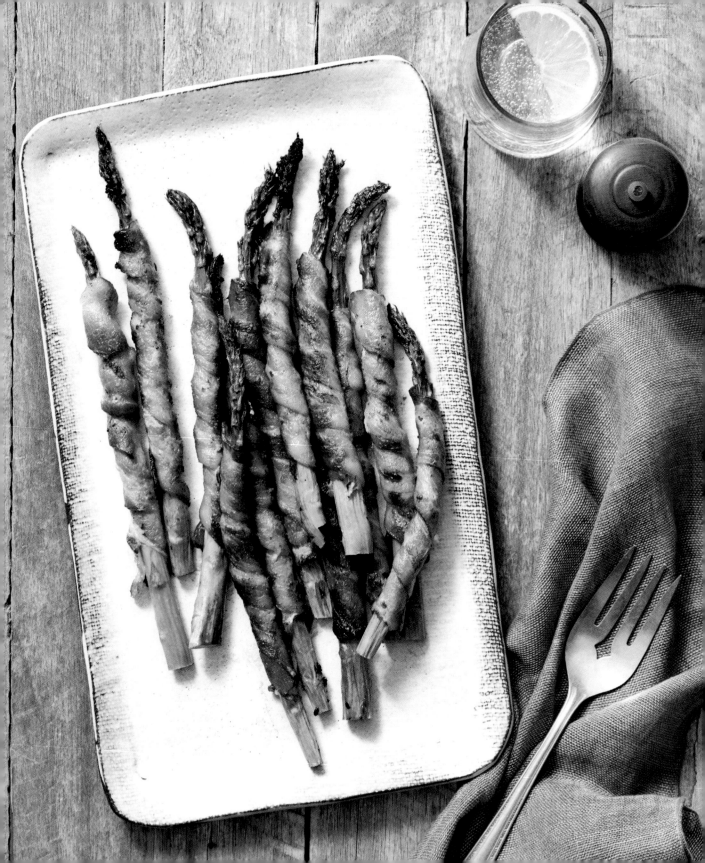

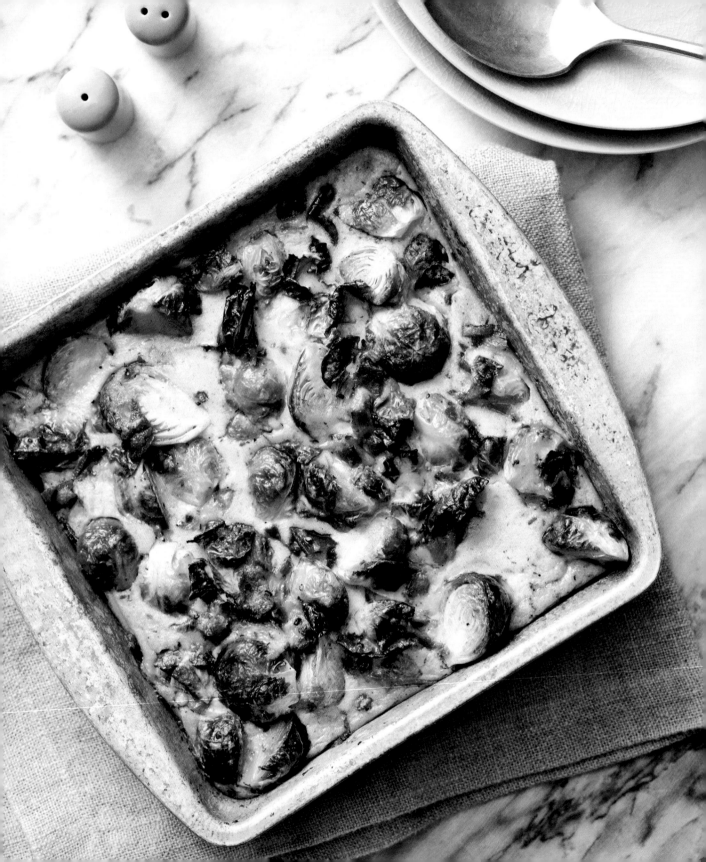

When you roast Brussels sprouts with bacon and cheese the result is a crave-able side dish that you'll want to make again and again.

BRUSSELS SPROUTS CASSEROLE

PREHEAT the oven to 400°F. Line a baking sheet with parchment paper or a silicone mat.

IN a medium bowl, toss the Brussels sprouts with the olive oil, salt, and pepper. Transfer to the prepared baking sheet and bake for 20 minutes, until tender. Transfer the Brussels sprouts to a baking dish and top with the crumbled bacon.

LOWER the oven temperature to 350°F. In a bowl, mix together the eggs, cheese, cream, rosemary, onion powder, garlic powder, and paprika until combined. Pour the egg mixture over the Brussels sprouts. Bake for 20 minutes, until bubbly. To get a nicely browned top, turn the oven to broil and broil for 5 minutes, watching carefully to make sure it doesn't burn.

NUTRITIONAL INFO (PER SERVING)
CALORIES 247, **FAT** 17.1 g, **PROTEIN** 15.6 g, **CARBS** 10 g, **FIBER** 3.1 g

MAKES 10 SERVINGS

~~~

1½ pounds Brussels sprouts, trimmed and cut in half

2 tablespoons extra-virgin olive oil

1 teaspoon salt

½ teaspoon black pepper

8 ounces sugar-free nitrite-free bacon, cooked and crumbled

2 large eggs, lightly beaten

1½ cups shredded cheddar and mozzarella mix

1 cup heavy cream

1 teaspoon minced fresh rosemary

1 teaspoon onion powder

1 teaspoon garlic powder

1 teaspoon paprika

It's amazing how three ingredients can turn into something so delicious! If you prefer bacon, go ahead and substitute it for the prosciutto. To secure the prosciutto around the cabbage you'll need toothpicks. Be sure to soak them in water for 30 minutes before using so they don't burn in the oven.

PROSCIUTTO-WRAPPED CABBAGE

MAKES 12 SERVINGS

~~~

1 head green cabbage

¼ teaspoon black pepper

6 ounces thinly sliced prosciutto

PREHEAT the oven to 375°F. Line a 9- by 13-inch baking sheet with parchment paper or a silicone mat.

CUT the cabbage into 1-inch-thick wedges and sprinkle with the pepper. Wrap each wedge with a slice of prosciutto. Secure with a toothpick.

PLACE the wedges on the prepared baking sheet and bake for 20 minutes. Turn over each wedge and continue to bake for 10 to 15 minutes longer, until the cabbage is tender and the prosciutto is crisp. Serve warm.

NUTRITIONAL INFO (PER SERVING)
CALORIES 60, **FAT** 5.6 g, **PROTEIN** 1.8 g, **CARBS** 0.5 g, **FIBER** 0.1 g

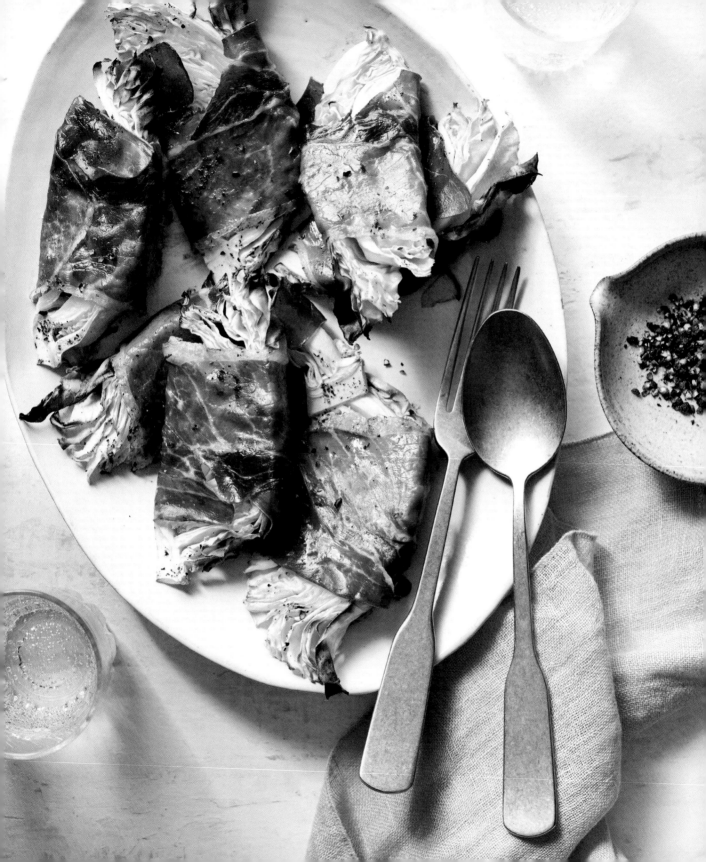

Here is another creamy side dish, this time featuring cauliflower and spinach. It goes really well with roasted meats like the Perfect Pork Tenderloin (page 128).

CAULIFLOWER-CREAMED SPINACH

PREHEAT the oven broiler.

BRING a large pot of water to a boil over high heat. Add the cauliflower and cook until tender, about 10 minutes. Using a slotted spoon, transfer the cauliflower to a food processor. Add the cream, butter, salt, and pepper and pulse until smooth.

HEAT the oil in a large cast-iron skillet over medium heat. Add the onion and cook, stirring, until translucent, 2 to 3 minutes. Add the spinach, mozzarella, nutmeg, and cloves and mix to combine. Add the cauliflower puree and cook, stirring, until heated through, 8 to 10 minutes.

PLACE the skillet under the broiler for 3 to 4 minutes, until the cheese has browned.

NUTRITIONAL INFO (PER SERVING)
CALORIES 153, **FAT** 8.6 g, **PROTEIN** 9.8 g, **CARBS** 14.2 g, **FIBER** 6.6 g

MAKES 6 SERVINGS

~~~

1 head cauliflower, cut into florets

2 tablespoons heavy cream

1 tablespoon butter

½ teaspoon salt

¼ teaspoon black pepper

1 tablespoon extra-virgin olive oil

1 small onion, diced

5 ounces baby spinach

½ cup shredded part-skim low-moisture mozzarella cheese

½ teaspoon ground nutmeg

Pinch ground cloves

Cooking frozen yellow squash in your microwave will save some time if you are in a super hurry. You will need two 12-ounce bags.

YELLOW SQUASH CASSEROLE

PREHEAT the oven to 350°F. Have a large baking dish ready.

FILL a 4-quart Dutch oven with water and bring to a boil over high heat. Add the squash and cook until tender, about 5 minutes. Drain the squash and return to the pot. Add the butter and mash the squash completely.

ADD the eggs, cream, stock, cream cheese, onion, parsley, Italian seasoning, garlic, salt, and pepper to the mashed squash. Pour the squash mixture into the baking dish and sprinkle with the cheddar. Bake for about 35 minutes, until the top is golden brown.

NOTE: *If you don't have Italian seasoning, you can make your own by combining equal amounts of dried basil, marjoram, oregano, rosemary, and thyme.*

NUTRITIONAL INFO (PER SERVING)
CALORIES 216, **FAT** 16.4 g, **PROTEIN** 8.3 g, **CARBS** 10.5 g, **FIBER** 1.8g

MAKES 8 SERVINGS

~~~

4 cups diced yellow squash

2 tablespoons butter

6 large eggs, beaten

½ cup heavy cream

¼ cup Stovetop Chicken Stock (page 67) or store-bought broth

4 tablespoons cream cheese, softened

1 tablespoon minced onion

1 tablespoon minced fresh parsley

1 teaspoon dried Italian seasoning (see Note)

1 teaspoon minced garlic

1 teaspoon salt

1 teaspoon black pepper

½ cup shredded cheddar cheese

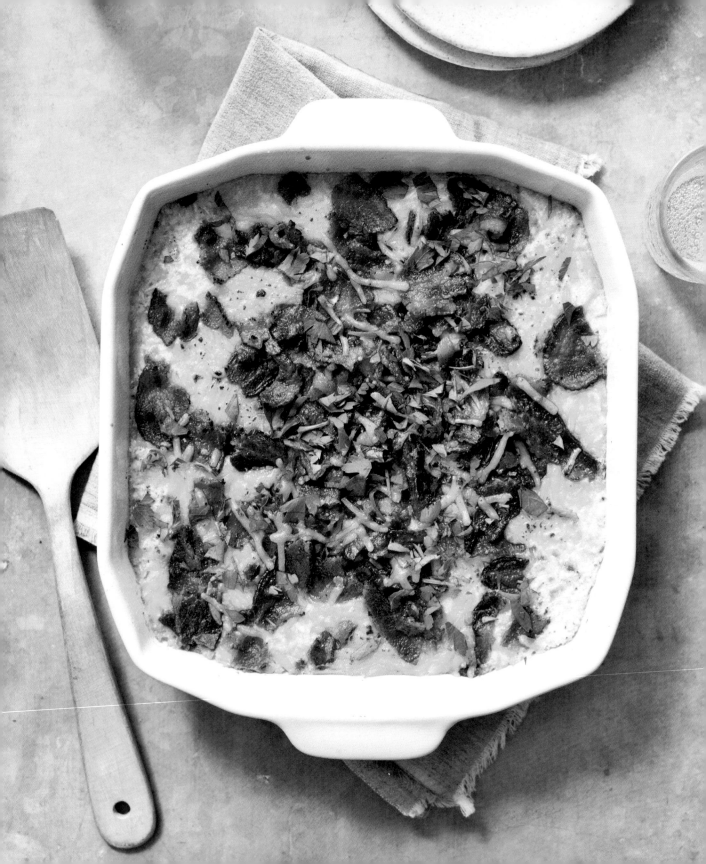

This is an excellent recipe for serving a large group like a family reunion or even on Thanksgiving.

CAULIFLOWER AND BACON AU GRATIN

PREHEAT the oven to 350°F. Spray a 9- by 13-inch baking dish with cooking spray.

IN a large skillet over medium heat, mix together the reserved bacon fat, cream, cream cheese, broth, and butter. Cook, stirring constantly, until the cream cheese has melted and mixed with the other ingredients. Add ½ cup of the cheddar cheese, the hot sauce, salt, pepper, and nutmeg and stir until blended.

PLACE the cauliflower in the prepared baking dish and spread out evenly. Pour the cheese mixture over the cauliflower. Sprinkle the remaining 1½ cups cheddar over the top and sprinkle the crumbled bacon over the cheese.

BAKE the casserole for 35 minutes, until it's golden brown on top and hot in the center. Sprinkle the parsley over the top just before serving.

NUTRITIONAL INFO (PER SERVING)
CALORIES 435, **FAT** 37.4 g, **PROTEIN** 20.3 g, **CARBS** 6 g, **FIBER** 1.2 g

MAKES 8 SERVINGS

- 10 slices sugar-free nitrite-free bacon, cooked and crumbled, bacon fat reserved
- 1 cup heavy cream
- 3 tablespoons cream cheese, cut into small pieces
- 3 tablespoons Pressure Cooker Bone Broth (page 65) or store-bought bone broth
- 2 tablespoons butter
- 2 cups shredded sharp cheddar cheese
- 1 teaspoon Frank's RedHot hot sauce
- 1 teaspoon salt
- 1 teaspoon black pepper
- ½ teaspoon ground nutmeg
- 1 (16-ounce) bag frozen cauliflower, thawed and cut into small pieces or riced
- 3 tablespoons minced fresh parsley

Sometimes it's hard when you can't have the little treats you used to eat before you started living a keto lifestyle. Made with cauliflower instead of potatoes, these keto-friendly tater tots will satisfy any craving you might have for fries with your burger. They are also good with eggs at breakfast instead of potato hash browns.

FAUXTATO TOTS

MAKES 4 SERVINGS

~~~~~

PREHEAT the oven to 375°F. Have a 24-cup mini muffin tin ready.

HEAT the frozen riced cauliflower in the microwave as instructed on the package. Drain and pat with paper towels to remove any excess liquid.

IN a large bowl, mix together the cauliflower, Parmesan, onion powder, garlic powder, salt, and pepper until fully combined. Add the olive oil and cheddar and mix together completely.

SPOON the mixture into the mini muffin tin, dividing evenly among the cups. Using a fork, press the mixture down into each cup. Bake for about 20 minutes, until the tots are golden brown. Serve hot.

STORE any leftovers in a covered container in the refrigerator for up to 2 days or in the freezer for up to 2 months. To reheat, defrost if frozen, and microwave for 30 to 45 seconds.

- 1 (12-ounce) bag frozen riced cauliflower
- 2 tablespoons grated Parmesan cheese
- ¼ teaspoon onion powder
- ¼ teaspoon garlic powder
- ½ teaspoon salt
- ¼ teaspoon black pepper
- 2 teaspoons extra-virgin olive oil
- ½ cup shredded cheddar cheese

NUTRITIONAL INFO (PER SERVING)
CALORIES 109, **FAT** 8.2 g, **PROTEIN** 5.7 g, **CARBS** 4.2 g, **FIBER** 1.7 g

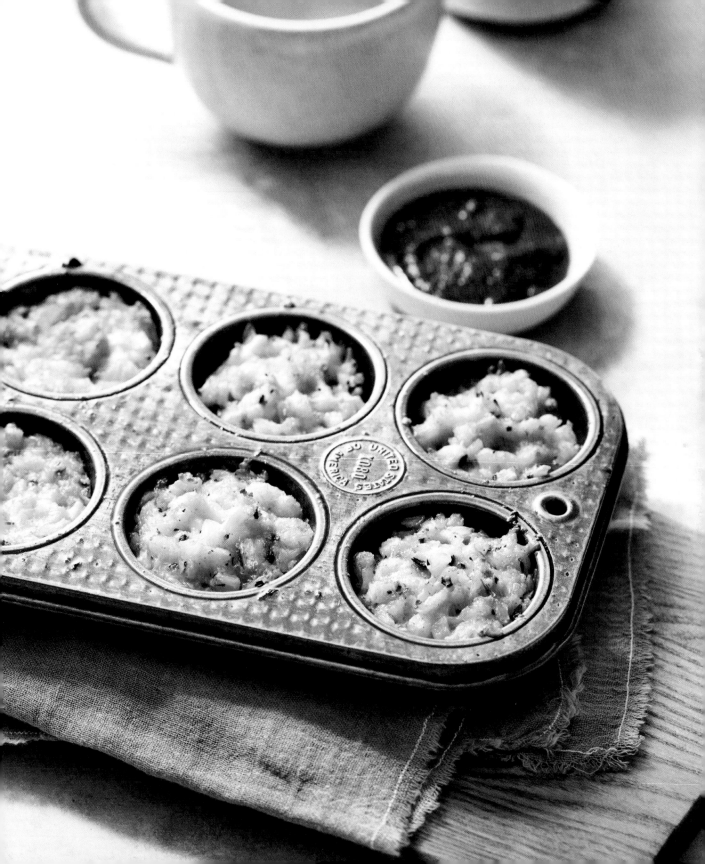

Here is a super tasty way to eat spaghetti squash. The creamy cheese sauce goes perfectly with the strands of squash, which look so pretty in their own squash bowls, garnished with parsley and green onions. This is a great dish to serve at a dinner party.

THREE-CHEESE GARLIC SPAGHETTI SQUASH

MAKES 4 SERVINGS

PREHEAT the oven to 400°F.

CUT the spaghetti squash in half lengthwise and scoop out the seeds. Place both halves cut side up on a baking sheet. Drizzle with the olive oil and rub it over the cut parts and the cavity. Sprinkle all over with the salt and pepper. Cover the squash and baking sheet with aluminum foil and roast for 40 minutes, until the squash is tender. Transfer the squash to a wire rack and let cool for at least 5 minutes, until it's cool enough to handle.

IN a large bowl, combine the eggs, cream, cheddar, Asiago, mozzarella, stock, garlic, and thyme.

USE a fork to scrape out the spaghetti squash noodles, reserving the "bowls." Add the noodles to the cheese mixture and mix together until fully combined. Set the spaghetti squash bowls on the baking sheet and divide the squash mixture between them. Bake for about 20 minutes, until all the cheese has melted and the top is golden brown.

TOP with the green onions and minced parsley and serve warm.

NOTE: *You can cut the baking time of this recipe by cooking the squash in a pressure cooker or microwave:*

For the pressure cooker, cut the squash in half, remove the seeds, and add to the pressure cooker with ½ cup chicken stock. Set on high and pressure cook for 11 minutes. Continue following the rest of the recipe.

1 large spaghetti squash

1 tablespoon extra-virgin olive oil

1 teaspoon salt

1 teaspoon black pepper

2 large eggs, lightly beaten

½ cup heavy cream

¼ cup shredded white cheddar cheese

¼ cup grated Asiago cheese

¼ cup shredded part-skim low-moisture mozzarella cheese

¼ cup Stovetop Chicken Stock (page 67) or store-bought chicken broth

1 tablespoon minced garlic

½ teaspoon minced fresh thyme

2 tablespoons sliced green onions

1 tablespoon minced fresh parsley

For the microwave, cut the squash in half, lay facedown in a shallow microwave-safe bowl, and add ½ cup chicken stock. Heat in the microwave oven on high until tender, 8 to 10 minutes, depending on the size of your squash and the power level of your microwave.

NUTRITIONAL INFO (PER SERVING)
CALORIES 236, **FAT** 19.4 g, **PROTEIN** 11 g, **CARBS** 5.5 g, **FIBER** 1 g

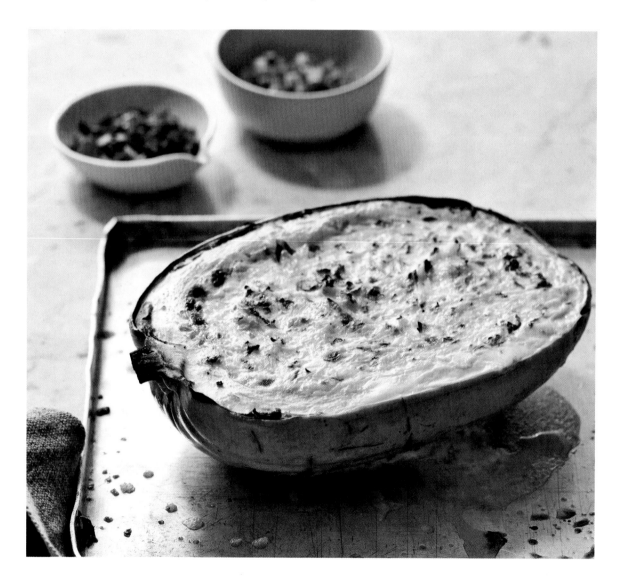

This is one of my most simple recipes, but it really tastes great. Try other cheeses like an Italian cheese blend, cheddar, or Monterey Jack. Serve as a side dish or as an appetizer or snack.

PARMESAN ZUCCHINI CRISPS

MAKES 4 SERVINGS

4 small zucchini

Salt and black pepper

1 cup shredded Parmesan cheese

Homemade Marinara Sauce (page 236) or store-bought low-sugar marinara sauce, for dipping

PREHEAT the oven to 425°F. Line a baking sheet with parchment paper or a silicone mat.

CUT the zucchini into ¼-inch-thick slices. Arrange on the prepared baking sheet and sprinkle with salt and pepper. Sprinkle the Parmesan evenly over the zucchini, making sure to cover each round.

BAKE for 15 to 20 minutes, checking at 10 minutes and then every 5 minutes, until the cheese turns golden brown.

SERVE with warmed marinara sauce on the side for dipping.

NUTRITIONAL INFO (PER SERVING)
CALORIES 109, **FAT** 5.9 g, **PROTEIN** 9.6 g, **CARBS** 5.4 g, **FIBER** 1.6 g

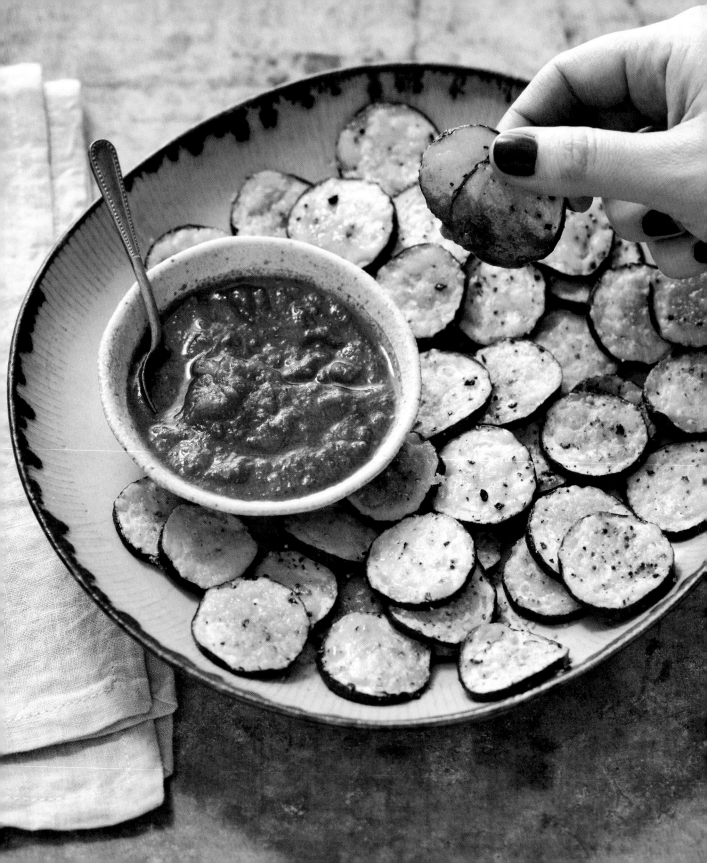

This is a good recipe in the summer when yellow squash and zucchini are everywhere and really fresh.

GREEN AND YELLOW SQUASH AU GRATIN

PREHEAT the oven to 350°F. Spray a baking dish with cooking spray.

IN a small skillet over medium heat, melt the butter. Add the onion and cook, stirring, until translucent, 3 to 5 minutes. Add 1 cup of the cheese, the cream, and garlic and stir to combine. Increase the heat to high and bring to a boil. Lower the heat and simmer until the cheese has melted and the sauce has thickened, about 10 minutes.

PLACE the zucchini and squash in the prepared baking dish. Pour the cheese sauce over the squash and sprinkle the remaining ½ cup cheese over the top.

BAKE for 25 to 30 minutes, until the cheese is golden brown and the squash is tender. Let cool for about 5 minutes before serving.

NUTRITIONAL INFO (PER SERVING)
CALORIES 242, **FAT** 22.2 g, **PROTEIN** 6.3 g, **CARBS** 5.6 g, **FIBER** 0.7 g

MAKES 8 SERVINGS

~~~

3 tablespoons butter

1 small onion, diced

1½ cups shredded cheese (such as Gouda, pepper Jack, or cheddar)

1 cup heavy cream

1 tablespoon minced garlic

2 small zucchini, thinly sliced

2 small yellow squash, thinly sliced

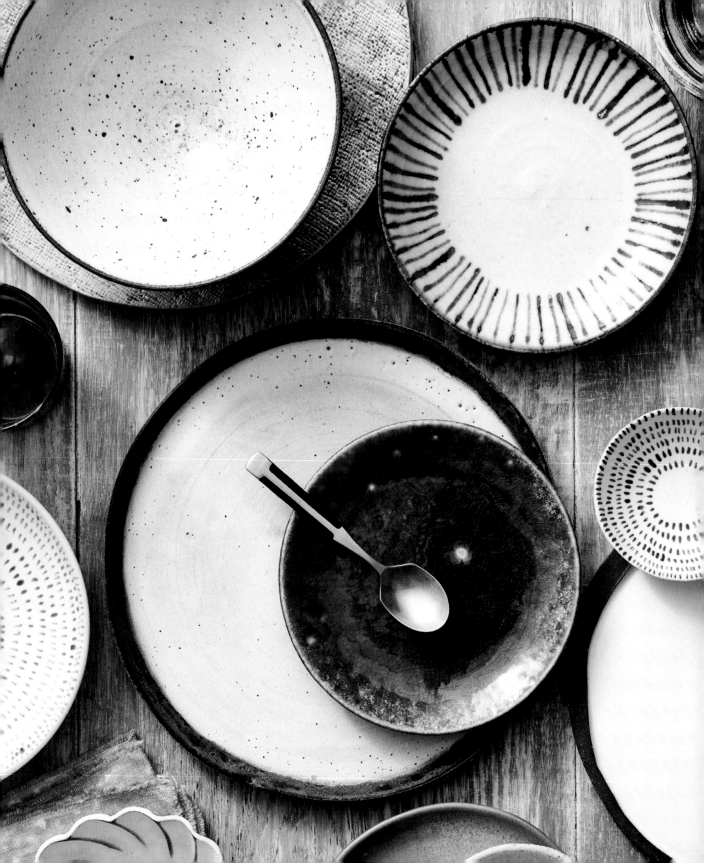

6

BREADS

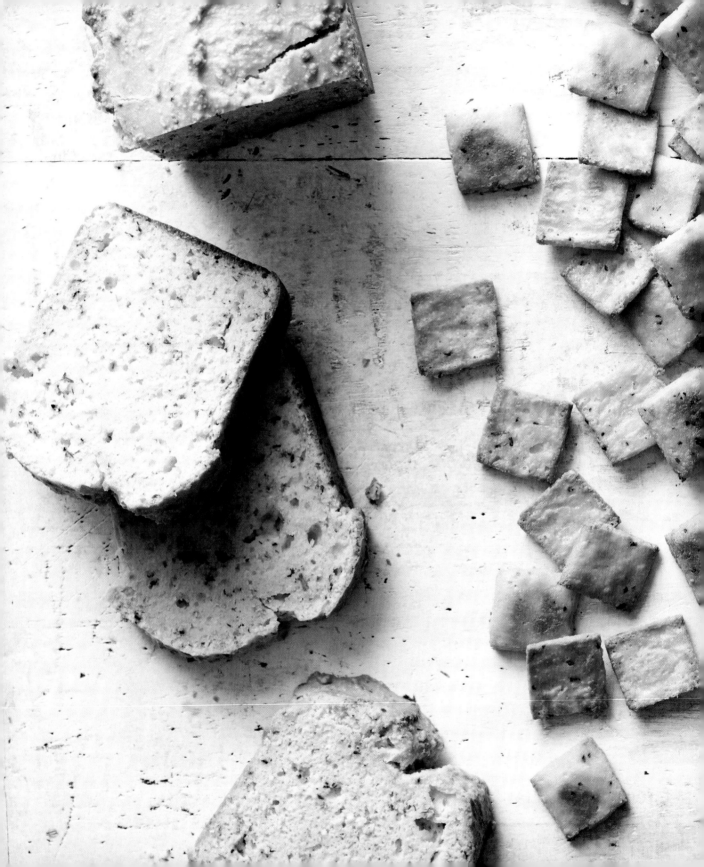

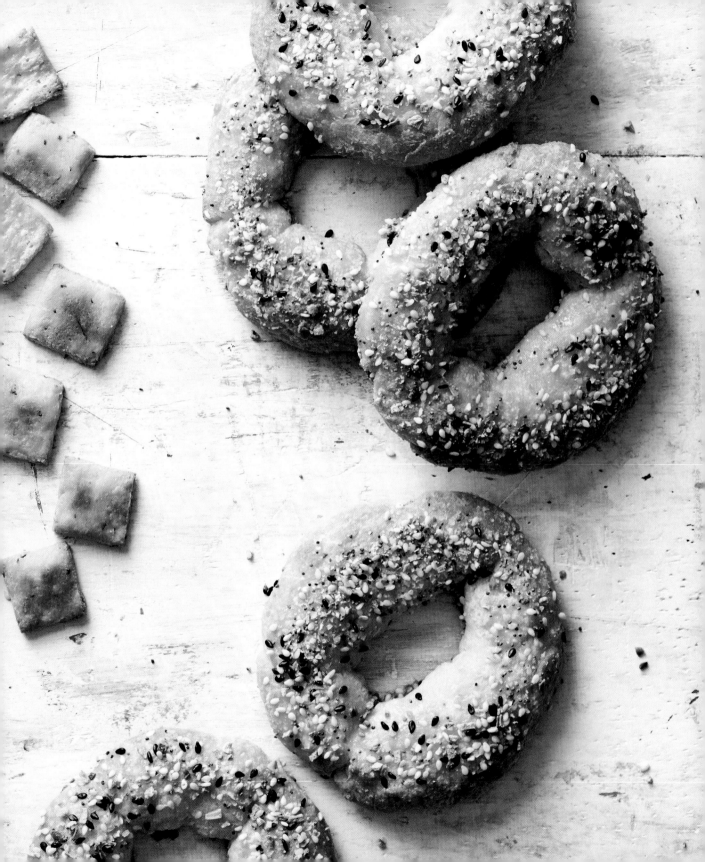

You can change the flavor of these biscuits by adding any seasonings you want. See the suggestions on page 186 for some of my favorite variations. You can also use a parchment paper–lined baking sheet instead of a muffin pan. Simply drop spoonfuls of dough on the pan and bake as instructed.

LOW-CARB BISCUITS

MAKES 12 SERVINGS

∿∿∿

- 1½ cups blanched almond flour
- 1 tablespoon baking powder
- ¼ teaspoon minced garlic
- ¼ teaspoon onion powder
- ¼ teaspoon salt
- 2 large eggs
- ½ cup sour cream
- 4 tablespoons butter, melted
- ½ cup shredded cheddar cheese

PREHEAT the oven to 450°F. Spray the cups of a 12-cup muffin pan with cooking spray.

IN a bowl, mix together the almond flour, baking powder, garlic, onion powder, and salt.

IN a separate bowl, whisk together the eggs, sour cream, and melted butter. Add the egg mixture to the flour mixture and stir with a spoon until combined. Add the shredded cheese and mix until combined.

SPOON the batter equally among the cups of the muffin pan. Bake for 10 to 13 minutes, until the tops start to brown.

NOTE: *If you coat the spoon with cooking spray before spooning batter into the muffin cups, it will slide off easily.*

NUTRITIONAL INFO (PER SERVING)
CALORIES 164, **FAT** 14.6 g, **PROTEIN** 5.8 g, **CARBS** 4.5 g, **FIBER** 1.5 g

(continued)

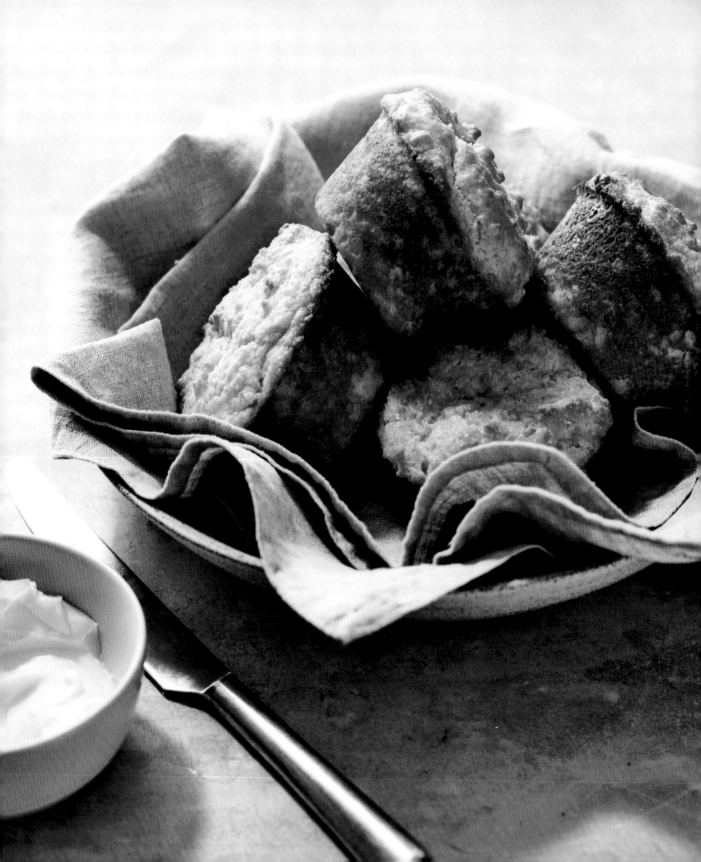

(Low-Carb Biscuits continued)

VARIATIONS

BACON-CHEDDAR: Leave out the garlic and onion powder and add ¾ cup cooked crumbled bacon along with the cheese.

JALAPEÑO-CHEDDAR: Leave out the garlic and onion powder and add ¼ cup chopped fresh jalapeño peppers along with the cheese.

CHIVE-CHEDDAR: Leave out the garlic and onion powder and add 3 tablespoons chopped fresh chives along with the cheese.

SPINACH-FETA: Leave out the garlic, onion powder, and cheddar cheese and add 1 cup fresh spinach and 1 cup feta cheese to the egg mixture.

ROSEMARY–GOAT CHEESE: Leave out the garlic, onion powder, and cheddar cheese and add 2 tablespoons chopped fresh rosemary and 1 cup goat cheese to the egg mixture.

BLUEBERRY–WHIPPED CREAM: Leave out the garlic, onion powder, and cheddar cheese and add 1 cup fresh blueberries before spooning into the muffin pan. Top the baked biscuits with whipped cream sweetened with stevia.

I call for blanched almond flour because it's made without the skins of the almonds. If you can't find it, simply use regular almond flour. Your hamburger buns will look a little darker but they will taste exactly the same.

HAMBURGER BUNS

MAKES 6 BUNS

~~~

PREHEAT the oven to 350°F. Have a nonstick hamburger bun pan or muffin top pan ready.

IN a microwave-safe bowl, heat the butter and cream cheese in the microwave oven until melted, 1 to 1½ minutes. Add the almond flour, baking powder, and eggs and mix until combined. Pour ¼ cup of the batter into each well of the pan. Sprinkle with sesame seeds, if using.

BAKE for 20 minutes, until golden brown. Let cool slightly before removing from the pan. Store in an airtight container for up to 4 days.

6 tablespoons butter, melted

2 ounces cream cheese, at room temperature

1¼ cups blanched almond flour

2 teaspoons baking powder

6 large eggs

Sesame seeds, optional

NUTRITIONAL INFO (PER SERVING)
CALORIES 231, **FAT** 14.2, **PROTEIN** 21.3 g, **CARBS** 7.8 g, **FIBER** 3.4 g

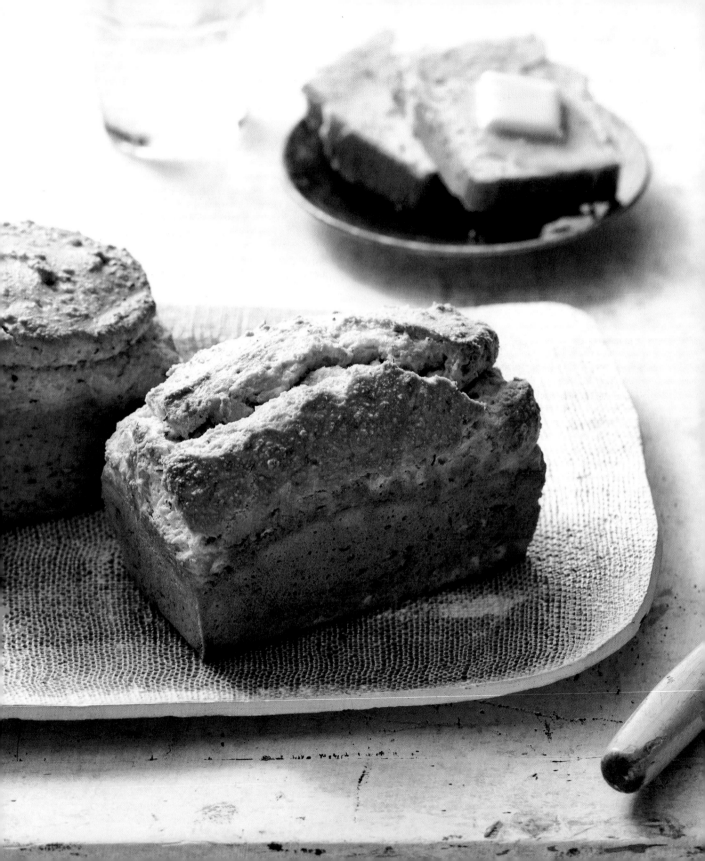

This recipe will become your go-to non-carb bread for making sandwiches at lunch or for toasting in the morning.

SAVORY KETO BREAD

PREHEAT the oven to 350°F. Spray 3 mini loaf pans (or 1 standard loaf pan) with cooking spray.

IN a mixing bowl, combine the butter and cream cheese and beat with an electric mixer until smooth. Add the parsley, rosemary, and sage and beat until fully combined. Add the eggs and continue to beat until smooth. With the mixer on low, beat in the almond flour, coconut flour, and baking powder. The batter will be thick.

FILL the mini loaf pans (or the single large pan) about halfway with the batter. Bake until the tops are golden brown and a toothpick inserted into the center of the loaf comes out clean, 35 minutes for mini loaves or 50 to 55 minutes for the larger loaf. Let cool for 5 minutes before turning out onto a wire rack to cool completely.

NUTRITIONAL INFO (PER SERVING)
CALORIES 163, **FAT** 14.7 g, **PROTEIN** 5.5 g, **CARBS** 4.2 g, **FIBER** 1.7 g

MAKES 24 SERVINGS

~~~

- 8 tablespoons butter
- 8 ounces cream cheese
- 2 tablespoons chopped fresh parsley
- 1 teaspoon dried rosemary
- 1 teaspoon dried sage
- 8 large eggs, at room temperature
- 2½ cups blanched almond flour
- ¼ cup coconut flour
- 1½ teaspoons baking powder

I often make this light and airy bread when I want a chicken salad sandwich, and I've got to say it makes an excellent peanut butter and jelly sandwich too.

CLOUD BREAD

MAKES 10 SERVINGS

PREHEAT the oven to 350°F. Line a baking sheet with parchment paper or a silicone mat.

IN a mixing bowl, beat the egg yolks and cream cheese with an electric mixer until fully blended. In a large bowl, with clean beaters, whisk the egg whites and baking powder with an electric mixer until they form peaks that hold their shape, about 5 minutes. Using a rubber spatula, carefully fold the egg yolk mixture into the whites, being careful to keep as much air in the mixture as possible. Do not overmix.

DROP about 10 spoonfuls of the batter onto the prepared baking sheet and use a spoon to spread each to about 4 inches wide and 1 inch thick. Sprinkle each with the rosemary, salt, and pepper. Bake for 15 to 20 minutes, until they are a light golden brown. Let cool and serve.

YOU can store the bread in a covered container in the refrigerator for up to one week. Reheat in the oven at 350°F for 2 to 3 minutes.

- 3 large eggs, separated
- 3 tablespoons cream cheese
- ¼ teaspoon baking powder
- ½ teaspoon dried rosemary
- ½ teaspoon salt
- ¼ teaspoon black pepper

NUTRITIONAL INFO (PER SERVING)
CALORIES 32, **FAT** 2.5 g, **PROTEIN** 2.1 g, **CARBS** 0.4 g, **FIBER** 0 g

VARIATION
To change up the flavors, feel free to sprinkle one of these seasonings over the batter before baking: everything bagel seasoning; roasted garlic and onion powder; Italian seasoning and Parmesan cheese; dried tarragon and cracked black pepper; cinnamon and melted butter; poppy seeds; sesame seeds; or basil and Parmesan cheese.

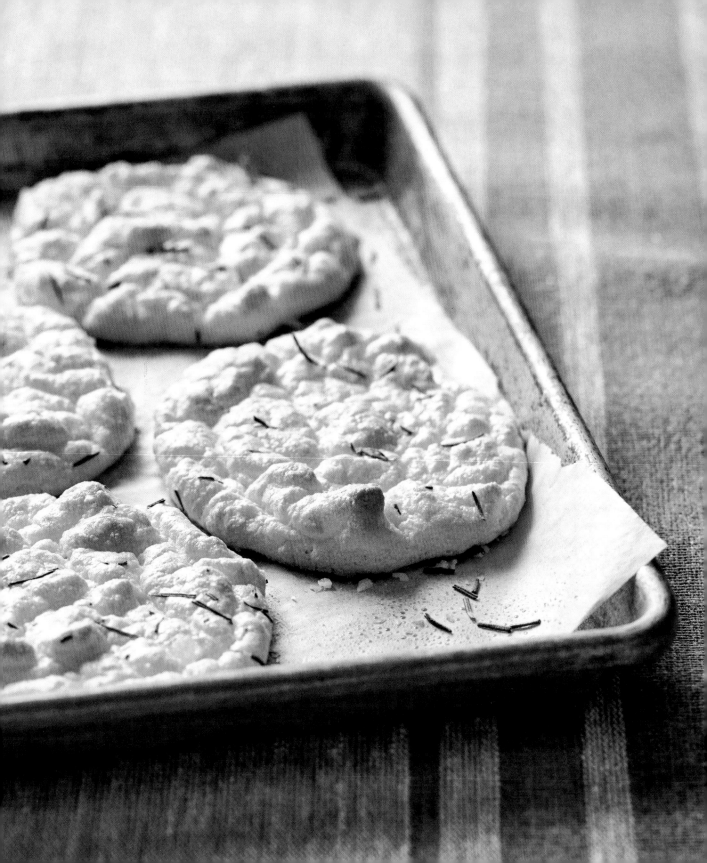

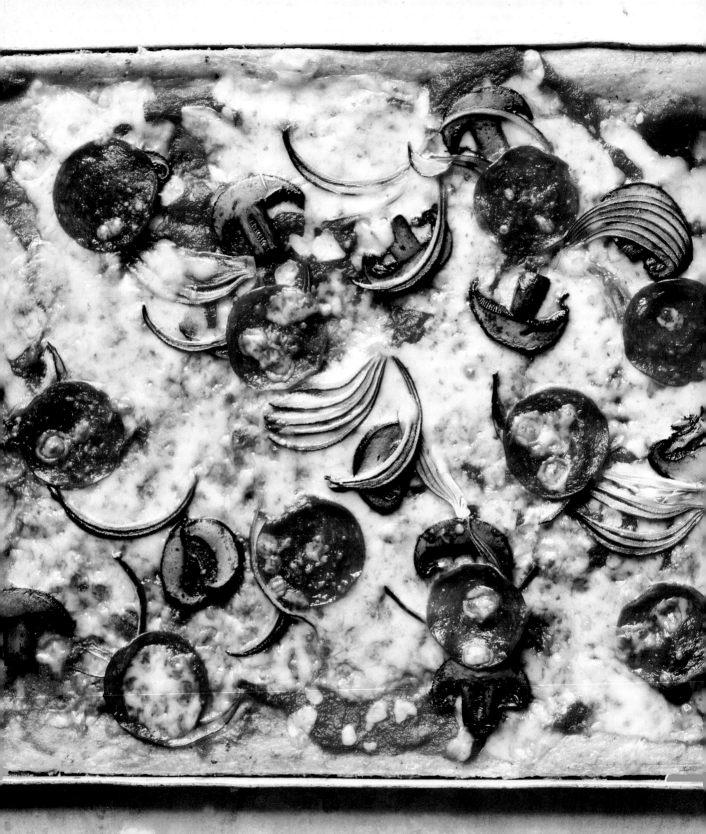

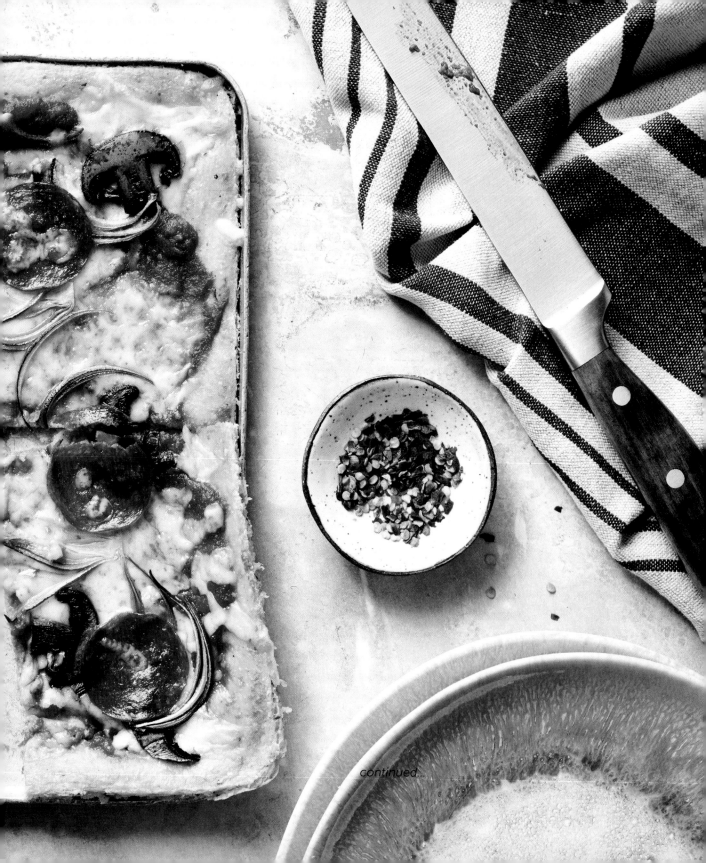

continued...

Pizza is one of the foods people are afraid they won't be allowed to eat when they start the keto program, so I knew I needed to share my recipe for pizza dough. No need to worry, everyone—pizza is still on the menu! And if you have kids, this is a nice recipe they can help you make. The dough freezes really nicely (see opposite); I usually make a triple batch, which makes six 12-inch pizzas.

KETO PIZZA DOUGH

MAKES 2 (12-INCH) PIZZA CRUSTS (8 SERVINGS)

PREHEAT the oven to 350°F. Have four large sheets of parchment paper and a baking sheet ready.

IN a microwave-safe bowl, heat the mozzarella, cream cheese, and almond flour in the microwave oven until the cheese melts, about 1 minute. Mix together until completely combined. Add the egg and the rosemary, if using, and mix until a sticky, stiff dough forms. Let cool for about 5 minutes.

DIVIDE the dough into two equal parts. Place one piece of dough onto one of the sheets of parchment paper and lay the other piece of parchment over the top. Using a rolling pin, roll out the dough into a 12-inch round. Slide the parchment with the dough onto the baking sheet. Discard the other piece of parchment.

ADD whatever toppings you like to the dough and bake for 12 to 15 minutes, until the crust turns a light golden brown. Slide the parchment with the baked pizza onto a wire rack and let cool for at least 5 minutes before cutting into slices with a large, sharp knife or a pizza cutter.

REPEAT to roll, top, and bake the second piece of dough.

- 1¾ cups shredded part-skim low-moisture mozzarella cheese
- 2 tablespoons cream cheese
- ¾ cup blanched almond flour
- 1 large egg
- 1 teaspoon dried rosemary, optional
- Toppings of choice, such as sausage, pepperoni, ham, spinach, mushrooms, onions, and/or green bell peppers

NUTRITIONAL INFO (PER SERVING)
CALORIES 126, **FAT** 9.8 g, **PROTEIN** 6.8 g, **CARBS** 3.9 g, **FIBER** 1.1 g

HOW TO FREEZE KETO PIZZA DOUGH

With a few frozen pizza crusts in your freezer, dinner is always less than an hour away.

Mix up the dough as instructed in the recipe. After rolling each piece of dough between two sheets of parchment, wrap each one individually in plastic wrap, stack them on top of each other, and store them flat in the freezer for up to 6 weeks.

To defrost the dough, set the frozen, rolled-out pizza dough on the counter at room temperature and let sit for about 20 minutes. Place the dough on a parchment-lined baking sheet, add whatever toppings you like, and bake as instructed in the recipe.

Yes, bagels are still allowed! Choose your favorite bagel flavoring and press into the dough before baking. Toast the bagels, spread on a little cream cheese, and you're in bagel heaven. Everything-but-the-bagel seasoning, a mixture of sesame seeds, poppy seeds, sea salt, dried garlic, and dried onions, is easy to find in the spice aisle at the grocery store.

KETO BAGELS

MAKES 6 BAGELS

~~~

PREHEAT the oven to 375°F. Line a baking sheet with parchment paper or a silicone mat. Have a sheet of parchment paper ready.

IN a microwave-safe bowl, heat the mozzarella and cream cheese in the microwave oven until melted, 1 to 1½ minutes. Add the almond flour, baking powder, salt, and egg and stir together until just combined.

TURN the dough out onto the piece of parchment paper and knead until all the dry ingredients have fully combined and the dough is no longer sticky. Work quickly when kneading; the dough will stiffen up as it cools and can become very hard to knead. If that happens, reheat the mixture in the microwave for 30 seconds and continue kneading.

DIVIDE the dough into six equal pieces. Roll each piece into a long, thick rope and press the ends together to form a circle. This dough will expand while baking, so be sure to leave a big enough opening in the center for a proper hole.

SPRINKLE the tops of the bagels with any seasonings you choose. Be sure to press the seasonings into the dough a bit to make sure they stick. Bake for 11 to 13 minutes, until golden brown. Let the bagels cool for about 5 minutes to firm up before you cut them.

2½ cups shredded part-skim low-moisture mozzarella cheese

3 tablespoons cream cheese, at room temperature

1¼ cups blanched almond flour

2 teaspoons baking powder

¼ teaspoon salt

1 large egg

OPTIONAL TOPPINGS

sesame seeds, poppy seeds, everything-but-the-bagel seasoning

NUTRITIONAL INFO (PER SERVING)
CALORIES 217, **FAT** 13.4 g, **PROTEIN** 20.2 g, **CARBS** 6.9 g, **FIBER** 3.3 g

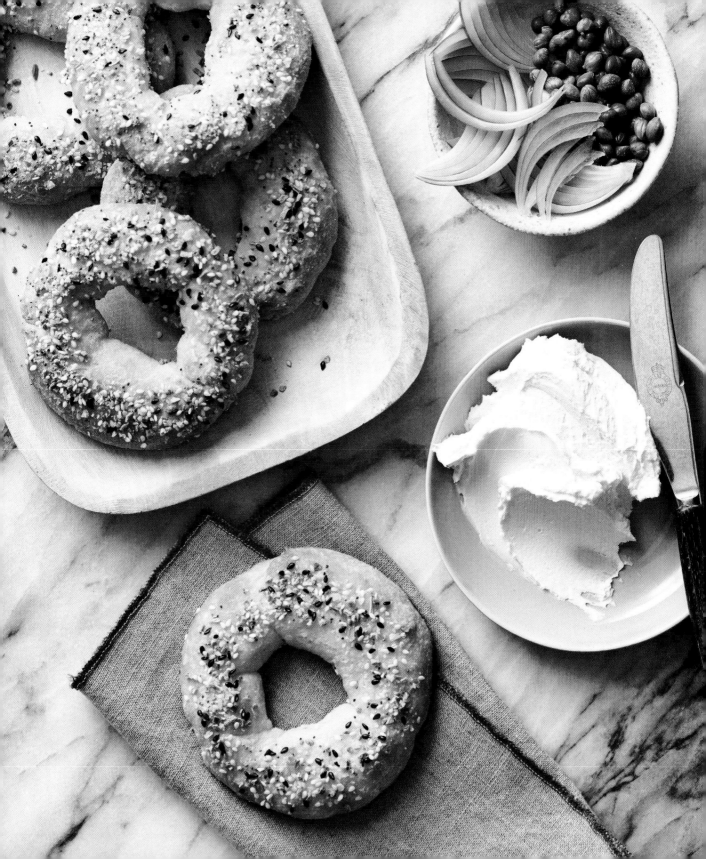

7

~~~~

DESSERT

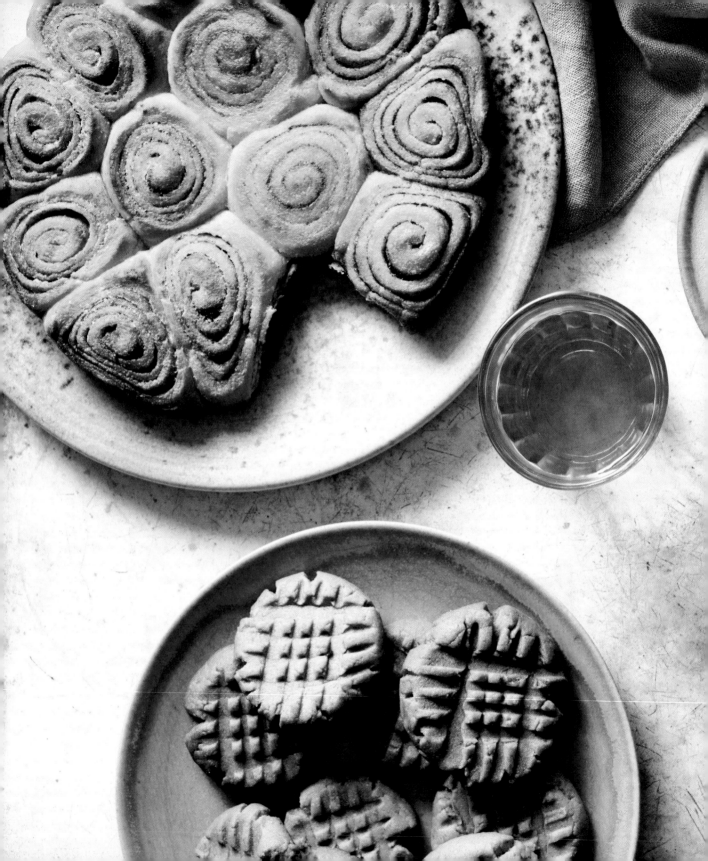

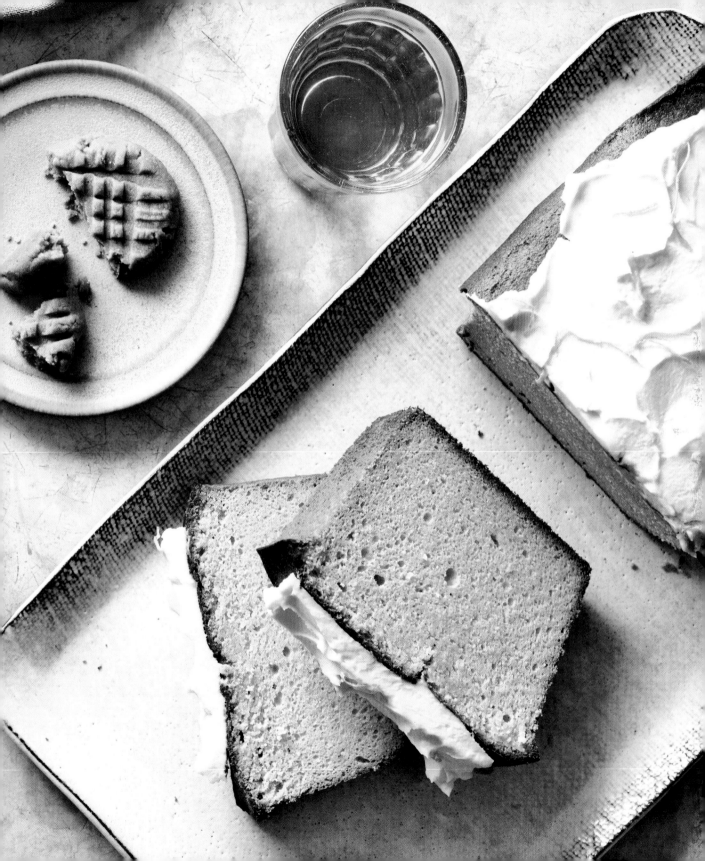

This is the basic recipe for Fat Bombs, a keto dieter's best friend. The main recipe is for the ever-popular cookie dough version, but I've also included a bunch of variations so you'll never get sick of them. I like to spoon the dough into silicone ice trays to refrigerate, because then the fat bombs are easy to portion out. But you can chill them in the bowl and just use a spoon to scoop out a portion whenever you want. By the way, the recipe will mix together much easier if all the ingredients are at room temperature.

CHOCOLATE CHIP COOKIE DOUGH FAT BOMBS

MAKES 24 SERVINGS

~~~

1 cup cream cheese, at room temperature

8 tablespoons butter, at room temperature

½ cup peanut butter or almond butter, at room temperature

10 drops liquid stevia or ⅓ cup Swerve confectioners' sweetener (see Note)

½ teaspoon vanilla extract

¾ cup Lily's stevia-sweetened dark chocolate chips (half a 9-ounce bag)

BEAT the cream cheese, butter, peanut butter, sweetener, and vanilla in a medium bowl with an electric mixer until smooth. Add the chocolate chips and use a spoon or a spatula to mix until combined.

IF you have silicone ice trays, spoon a 1-tablespoon portion of dough into each cavity and refrigerate for at least 30 minutes before serving. If you don't have trays, simply cover the bowl with plastic wrap, place it into the refrigerator, and scoop out portions as needed.

FAT bombs can be stored in a covered container in the refrigerator for up to 2 weeks.

NOTE: *Liquid stevia is my favorite sweetener for fat bombs because I can easily adjust the sweetness by increasing or decreasing the number of drops, and it doesn't interfere with the lovely smooth texture.*

I tried using erythritol, and it tasted great but I didn't like the slightly gritty texture. You can use Swerve, which combines with the ingredients better than erythritol, but I still think the liquid stevia version has better flavor.

NUTRITIONAL INFO (PER 1 TABLESPOON)
CALORIES 83, **FAT** 8.2 g, **PROTEIN** 1.7 g, **CARBS** 3.2 g, **FIBER** 0.5 g

(continued)

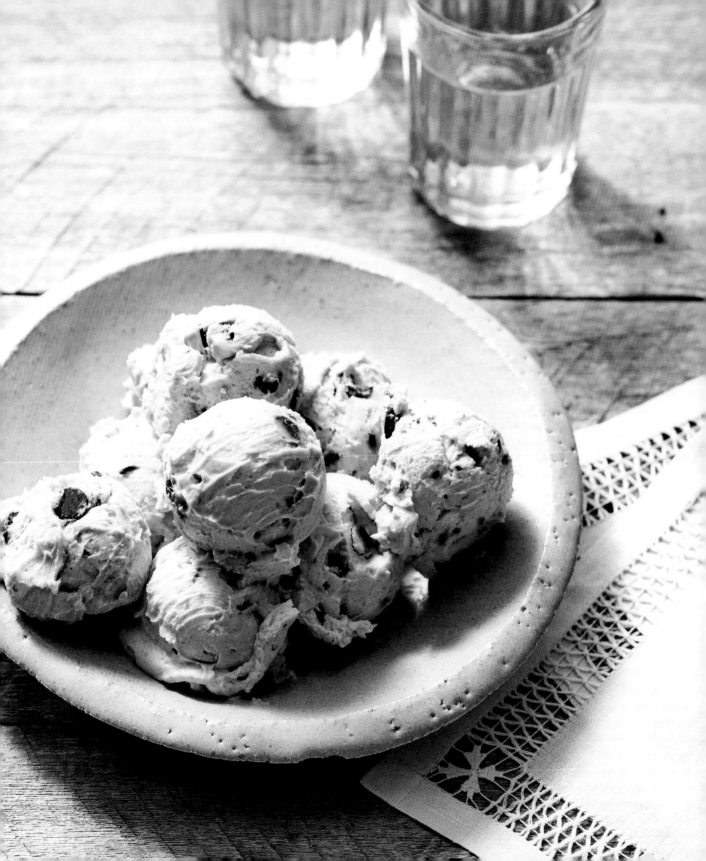

(Chocolate Chip Cookie Dough Fat Bombs continued)

VARIATIONS

CHOCOLATE CHIP LOVERS: Leave out the peanut butter. The texture changes a bit but they taste amazing.

STRAWBERRY CHEESECAKE: Leave out the peanut butter and chocolate chips. Add 1 cup chopped fresh strawberries.

RASPBERRY CHEESECAKE: Leave out the peanut butter and chocolate chips. Add 1 cup fresh raspberries.

RASPBERRY-LEMON CHEESECAKE: Leave out the peanut butter and chocolate chips. Add 1 cup fresh raspberries, 1 tablespoon grated lemon zest, and 2 tablespoons fresh lemon juice.

CHOCOLATE CHEESECAKE: Add 4 tablespoons unsweetened cocoa powder and ¼ teaspoon salt. Chop up the chocolate chips and roll the chocolate cheesecake balls in the chopped chocolate before chilling.

BLUEBERRY CHEESECAKE: Leave out the peanut butter and chocolate chips. Add 1 cup fresh blueberries.

BLUEBERRY-LEMON CHEESECAKE: Leave out the peanut butter and chocolate chips. Add 1 cup fresh blueberries, 1 tablespoon grated lemon zest, and 2 tablespoons fresh lemon juice.

LEMON CHEESECAKE: Leave out the peanut butter and chocolate chips. Add 1 tablespoon grated lemon zest and 2 tablespoons fresh lemon juice.

RASPBERRY-LEMON CHEESECAKE: Leave out the peanut butter and chocolate chips. Add 1 cup fresh raspberries, 1 tablespoon grated lemon zest, and 2 tablespoons fresh lemon juice.

You are going to love this fudge. Smooth and really chocolatey, it's hard to believe it's OK to eat this on the diet. Package them up in a box and tie with a pretty ribbon and you'll have a nice hostess gift.

LOW-CARB CHOCOLATE FUDGE

HAVE an 8-inch square pan ready.

IN a saucepan over medium-low heat, melt the chocolate chips and butter, stirring, until combined. Remove from the heat.

IN a bowl, beat the cream cheese with an electric mixer. Add the melted chocolate and butter mixture and beat until fully combined, about 2 minutes. Add the sweetener and continue to beat on low until fully combined.

POUR the mixture into the pan. If you like, arrange pecan halves decoratively over the top.

COVER and place the pan in the freezer until it firms up, at least 15 minutes. Cut the fudge into 1-inch squares.

STORE in a covered container in the refrigerator for up to 7 days or in the freezer for up to 2 months.

MAKES 32 SERVINGS

~~~

1½ cups Lily's stevia-sweetened dark chocolate chips (one 9-ounce bag)

8 tablespoons butter

8 ounces cream cheese

¼ cup Swerve confectioners' sweetener

32 pecan halves, optional

NUTRITIONAL INFO (PER SERVING)
CALORIES 51, **FAT** 5.3 g, **PROTEIN** 0.5 g, **CARBS** 0.9 g, **FIBER** 0 g

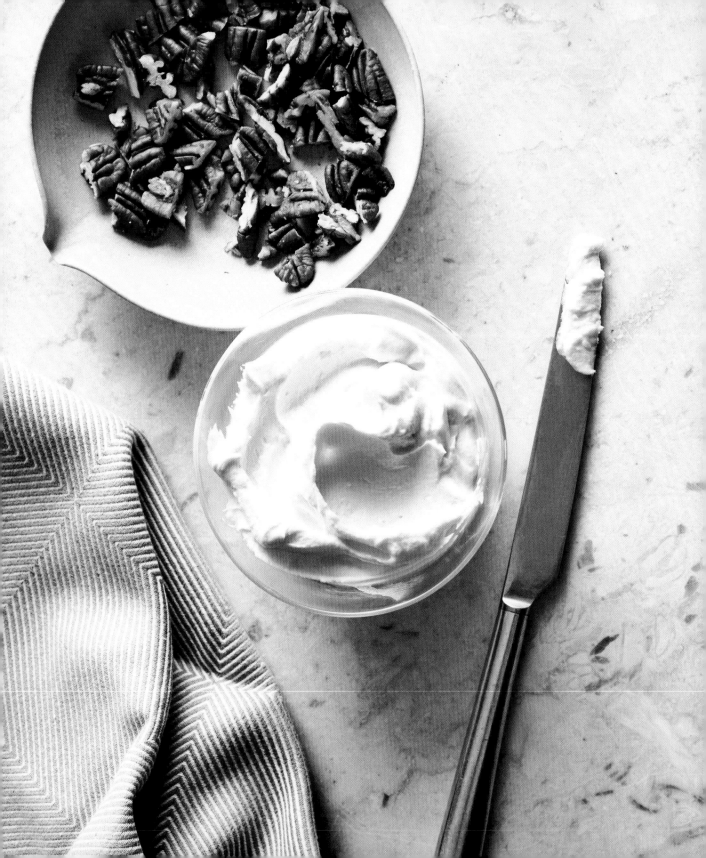

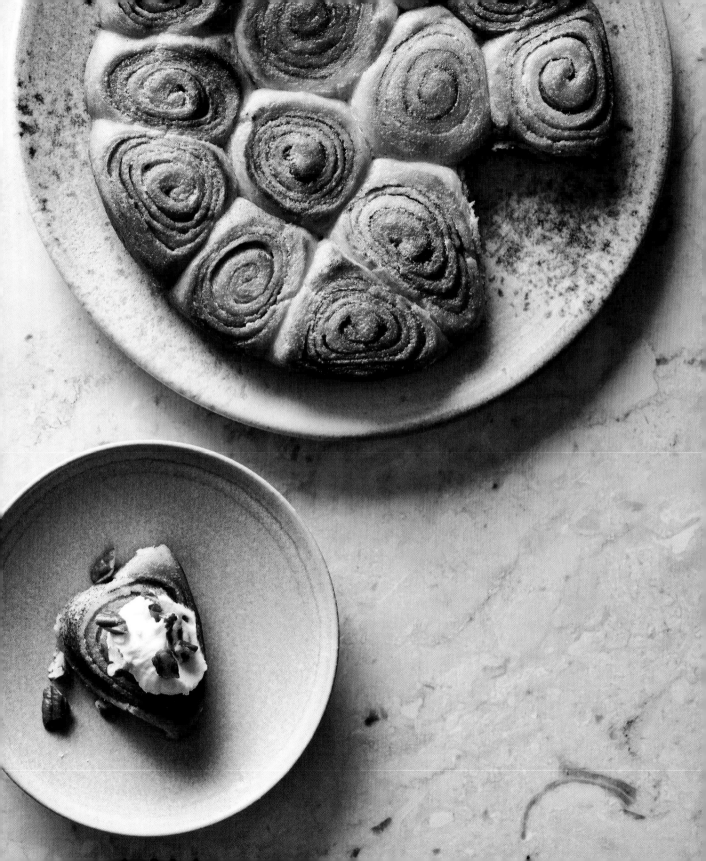

These will make your kitchen smell so good! And with their drippy cream cheese frosting you'll have a hard time eating just one.

CINNAMON ROLLS

PREHEAT the oven to 350°F. Have a large sheet of parchment paper ready. Line a baking sheet with parchment paper.

FOR THE DOUGH

IN a microwave-safe bowl, heat the mozzarella and cream cheese in the microwave oven until melted, 1 minute. Add the egg, almond flour, and baking powder and stir until smooth. The dough will be very sticky at this point.

TRANSFER the dough onto the parchment paper and knead until the ingredients are fully mixed in. Sprinkle a little bit of almond flour on the dough if it becomes too sticky.

SPRINKLE some of the almond flour onto the dough and a rolling pin and roll out the dough to a 10- by 15-inch rectangle. Brush the butter evenly over the rolled-out dough. Sprinkle the stevia and cinnamon evenly over the dough.

STARTING on a longer side, roll up the dough as tightly as possible. Using a very sharp knife, cut the dough into 15 equal slices. Place the slices, cut side up, on the prepared baking sheet.

BAKE for 20 minutes, until the rolls are golden brown. Transfer to a baking rack to cool for 5 to 10 minutes.

FOR THE FROSTING

BEAT the cream, cream cheese, sweetener, and vanilla in a bowl with an electric mixer on high speed for 4 to 5 minutes, until smooth.

SPREAD the frosting on the cinnamon rolls. Sprinkle with chopped pecans, if using, and serve warm.

MAKES 15 SERVINGS

~~~

CINNAMON ROLL DOUGH

2 cups shredded part-skim low-moisture mozzarella cheese

3 tablespoons cream cheese

1 large egg

¾ cup blanched almond flour, plus more for sprinkling

1 teaspoon baking powder

1 tablespoon butter, melted

1 tablespoon powdered stevia or Swerve confectioners' sweetener

1 teaspoon ground cinnamon

CREAM CHEESE FROSTING

2 tablespoons heavy cream

2 tablespoons cream cheese

1 tablespoon Swerve confectioners' sweetener

¼ teaspoon vanilla extract

1 cup chopped pecans, optional

NUTRITIONAL INFO (PER SERVING)
CALORIES 98, **FAT** 8 g, **PROTEIN** 4.6 g, **CARBS** 3.5 g, **FIBER** 0.7 g

Coffee cake doesn't usually contain strawberries, but when I tested this recipe, I knew I had discovered something really good.

STRAWBERRY CRUMBLE COFFEE CAKE

PREHEAT the oven to 350°F. Spray a 9-inch square baking dish with cooking spray.

FOR THE CAKE

IN a mixing bowl, beat the butter and sweetener together with an electric mixer for 3 to 4 minutes, until smooth. Add the eggs and vanilla and continue to beat until incorporated. Add the almond flour, coconut flour, baking powder, xanthan gum, and salt and beat on low until smooth. Add the coconut milk and beat until smooth.

SPREAD the dough evenly in the baking dish. Sprinkle the chopped strawberries over the batter. Set aside.

FOR THE TOPPING

IN a mixing bowl, beat the cream cheese with an electric mixer until light and fluffy, 1 to 2 minutes. Add the egg and sweetener and continue beating until smooth.

POUR the cream cheese topping over the top of the strawberries. Bake the cake for 20 minutes, until a toothpick inserted into the center comes out clean.

FOR THE STREUSEL

MEANWHILE, place the butter in a microwave-safe bowl and heat in the microwave oven until melted, about 20 seconds. Stir in the almond flour, coconut flour, sweetener, lemon zest, and vanilla until fully combined.

(continued)

MAKES 12 SERVINGS

~~~

COFFEE CAKE

6 tablespoons butter

½ cup Swerve confectioners' sweetener

2 large eggs

2 teaspoons vanilla extract

1 cup blanched almond flour

¼ cup coconut flour

2 teaspoons baking powder

¼ teaspoon xanthan gum

¼ teaspoon salt

½ cup unsweetened coconut milk

1½ cups chopped strawberries

CREAM CHEESE TOPPING

3 ounces cream cheese

1 large egg

1 tablespoon Swerve confectioners' sweetener

STREUSEL

3 tablespoons butter

1 cup blanched almond flour

1 teaspoon coconut flour

3 tablespoons Swerve confectioners' sweetener

1 teaspoon grated lemon zest

½ teaspoon vanilla extract

(Strawberry Crumble Coffee Cake continued)

REMOVE the cake from the oven and top evenly with the streusel. Bake for another 15 to 20 minutes, until a toothpick comes out clean when inserted into the center of the cake. Cut into 12 pieces and serve, or store in a covered container in the refrigerator for up to 4 days; reheat in the microwave for 20 to 30 seconds or enjoy cold.

NUTRITIONAL INFO (PER SERVING)
CALORIES 262, **FAT** 23.6 g, **PROTEIN** 6.9 g, **CARBS** 13.4 g, **FIBER** 3.7 g

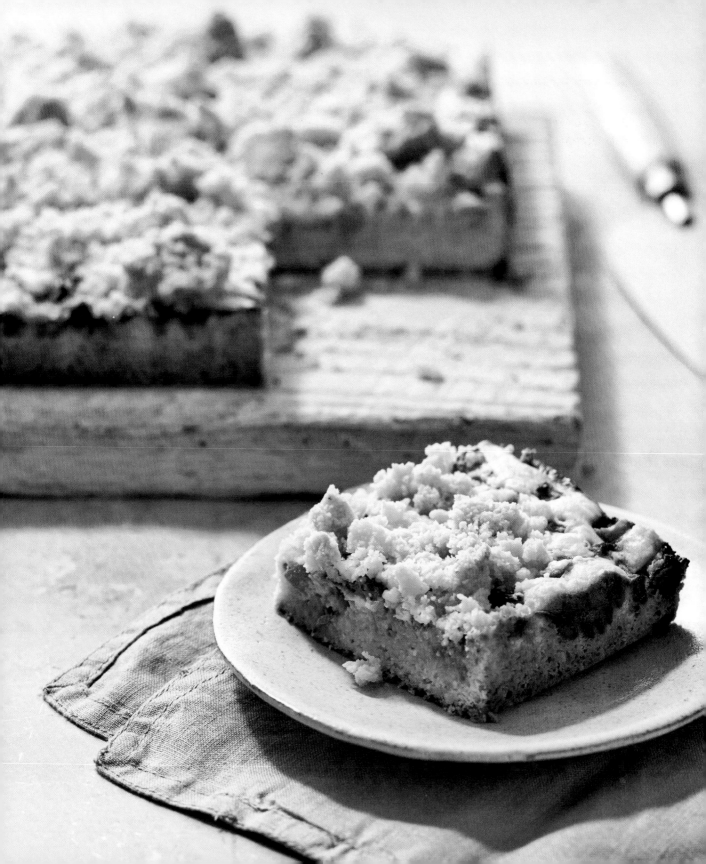

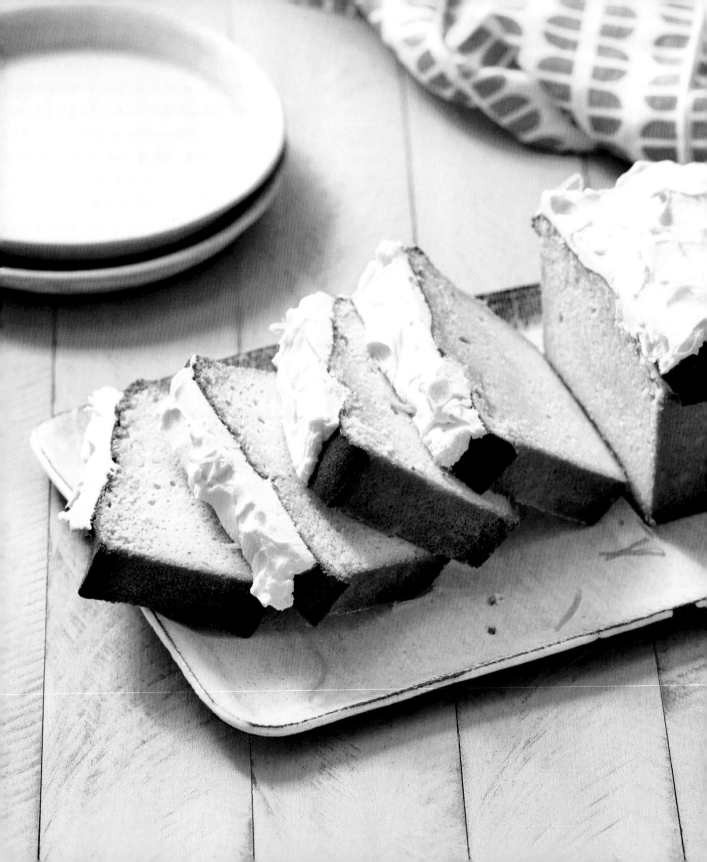

Serve slices of this sweet lemon pound cake after a dinner party or with afternoon tea.

LEMON POUND CAKE

MAKES 16 SERVINGS

~~~

PREHEAT the oven to 350°F. Spray two mini loaf pans or one standard loaf pan with cooking spray.

IN a mixing bowl, beat the butter and sweetener with an electric mixer until smooth, 2 to 3 minutes. Add the cream cheese and continue to beat until smooth. Add the eggs, vanilla, lemon zest, and lemon extract and continue to beat until thoroughly combined.

ADD the almond flour, baking powder, and salt and beat until smooth. Divide the batter equally between the two mini loaf pans, or pour it all into the larger pan.

BAKE for about 35 minutes for mini loaves or about 60 minutes for a larger loaf, until a toothpick inserted in the center of a loaf comes out clean. Let cool completely before frosting.

FOR THE LEMON FROSTING

BEAT the cream cheese, sweetener, cream, and vanilla in a bowl with an electric mixer for 5 to 7 minutes, until smooth.

USING a knife or a spatula, frost the top of the cake(s) with the frosting.

CUT into slices and serve, or store in a covered container in the refrigerator for up to 4 days; reheat in the microwave for 20 to 30 seconds or enjoy cold.

8 tablespoons butter

1½ cups Swerve confectioners' sweetener

8 ounces cream cheese

8 large eggs, at room temperature

1½ teaspoons vanilla extract

1 tablespoon grated lemon zest

1 teaspoon lemon extract

2½ cups blanched almond flour

1½ teaspoons baking powder

½ teaspoon salt

LEMON FROSTING

4 ounces cream cheese

¼ cup Swerve confectioners' sweetener

3 tablespoons heavy cream

½ teaspoon vanilla extract

NUTRITIONAL INFO (PER SERVING)
CALORIES 273, **FAT** 25.2 g, **PROTEIN** 8.3 g, **CARBS** 10.7 g, **FIBER** 1.9 g

This cake is a perfect afternoon treat, plus it has some healthy benefits. Collagen helps to improve gut health, build muscle, and burn fat, and it's also known to reduce signs of aging. I try to sneak it into recipes when I can because you won't even taste it. You can buy collagen online.

BLUEBERRY POUND CAKE

~~~

PREHEAT the oven to 350°F. Line the bottom of an 8- by 4-inch loaf pan with parchment paper. Spray the pan with cooking spray.

IN a bowl, combine the almond flour, coconut flour, collagen, baking powder, and salt and stir to combine.

IN a mixing bowl, beat the eggs and vanilla with an electric mixer on high until light and fluffy, about 1 minute. Add the almond milk, sour cream, melted butter, and lemon zest and beat until combined. Add the dry ingredients in thirds, beating on low between each addition, until smooth. With a spatula, gently fold in the blueberries.

POUR the batter into the prepared loaf pan and bake for 55 to 60 minutes, until the top is golden brown and a toothpick inserted into the center comes out clean. Let cool completely. Cut into slices and serve, or store in a covered container in the refrigerator for up to 4 days; reheat in the microwave for about 30 seconds or enjoy cold.

1½ cups blanched almond flour

¼ cup coconut flour

2 tablespoons collagen protein powder

1 teaspoon baking powder

¼ teaspoon salt

3 large eggs

1 teaspoon vanilla extract

1 cup almond milk

¼ cup sour cream

4 tablespoons butter, melted

1 teaspoon grated lemon zest

1 cup fresh blueberries

NUTRITIONAL INFO (PER SERVING)
CALORIES 127, **FAT** 13.2 g, **PROTEIN** 5.7 g, **CARBS** 7.2 g, **FIBER** 2.6 g

The combination of fiber, whey, and xanthan gum gives these frozen treats an amazing creamy texture! If you don't have these ingredients, you can still make the recipe—you won't get the same texture but they will still taste great.

CREAMY BLUEBERRY ICE POPS

COMBINE ¾ cup water and all the ingredients in a blender and puree until completely combined. Pour into six 4-ounce popsicle molds and freeze for at least 8 hours before serving.

NUTRITIONAL INFO (PER SERVING)
CALORIES 47, **FAT** 1.3 g, **PROTEIN** 4.8 g, **CARBS** 8.1 g, **FIBER** 0.3 g

MAKES 8 SERVINGS

~~~

½ cup coconut milk

½ cup blueberries

¼ cup monkfruit powdered sweetener

¼ cup sour cream

2 tablespoons whey protein

1 teaspoon unflavored fiber

¼ teaspoon xanthan gum

Nature's Eats makes a blanched almond flour that I use for the cakes and cupcakes that I want to be as light colored as possible. But if you can't find it, use regular almond flour—it will taste just as good. Raspberry and lemon are two flavors that were born to be together and these cupcakes prove the point.

RASPBERRY-LEMON CUPCAKES

MAKES 16 SERVINGS

PREHEAT the oven to 350°F. Coat 16 cupcake liners with cooking spray and place in the cups of two cupcake pans.

IN a mixing bowl, combine the almond flour, coconut flour, baking powder, baking soda, xanthan gum, and salt and whisk together until blended. Set aside.

IN another mixing bowl, beat together the stevia, butter, and the 4 eggs with an electric mixer until creamed. Add the cream, vinegar, raspberry extract, lemon extract, and lemon zest and continue to beat until combined.

ADD the dry ingredients to the wet ingredients and mix thoroughly. Fold the raspberries into the batter. Set aside.

IN a separate bowl, with clean beaters, beat the 2 egg whites until they form stiff peaks. Carefully fold the whites into the batter until incorporated.

SPOON the batter into the prepared cupcake liners, filling each two-thirds full. Tap the tray on the counter to release any trapped air bubbles and level out the batter. Bake for 25 minutes, until golden brown. Cool on a wire rack, although they are delicious warm. Store in a covered container in the refrigerator for up to 4 days; reheat in the microwave for 20 to 30 seconds or enjoy cold.

- 2 cups blanched almond flour
- ⅔ cup coconut flour
- 1 tablespoon baking powder
- 1 teaspoon baking soda
- 1 teaspoon xanthan gum
- ½ teaspoon pink Himalayan salt
- 1 cup Pyure organic powdered stevia (Bakeable Blend)
- 8 tablespoons unsalted butter, softened
- 4 large eggs plus 2 egg whites, at room temperature
- ½ cup heavy cream
- 1 teaspoon apple cider vinegar
- 1 teaspoon raspberry extract
- 1 teaspoon lemon extract
- ½ teaspoon grated lemon zest
- 1 cup fresh raspberries

NUTRITIONAL INFO (PER SERVING)
CALORIES 203, **FAT** 17.2 g, **PROTEIN** 6.4 g, **CARBS** 9.9 g, **FIBER** 3.8 g

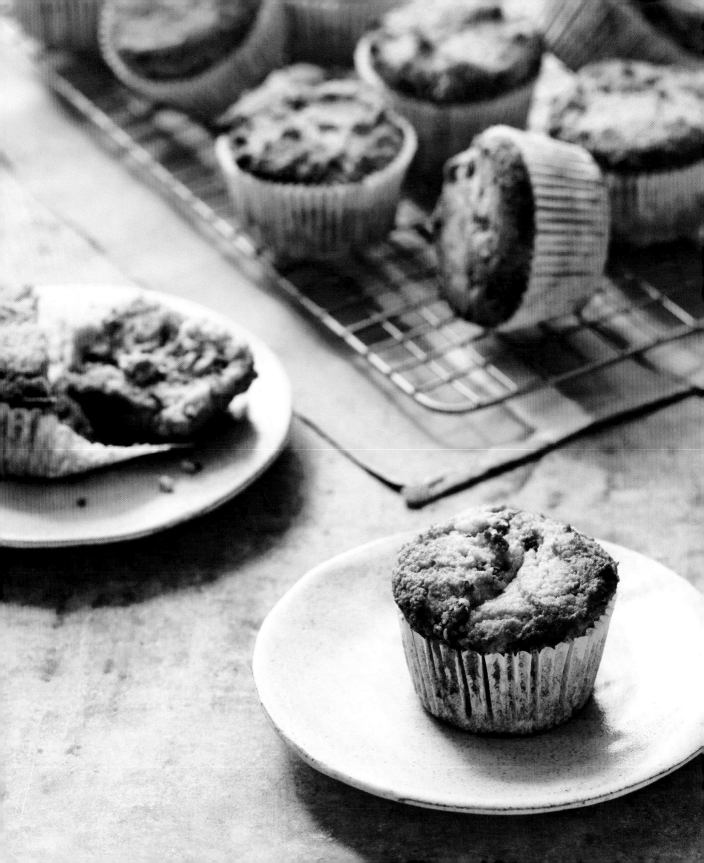

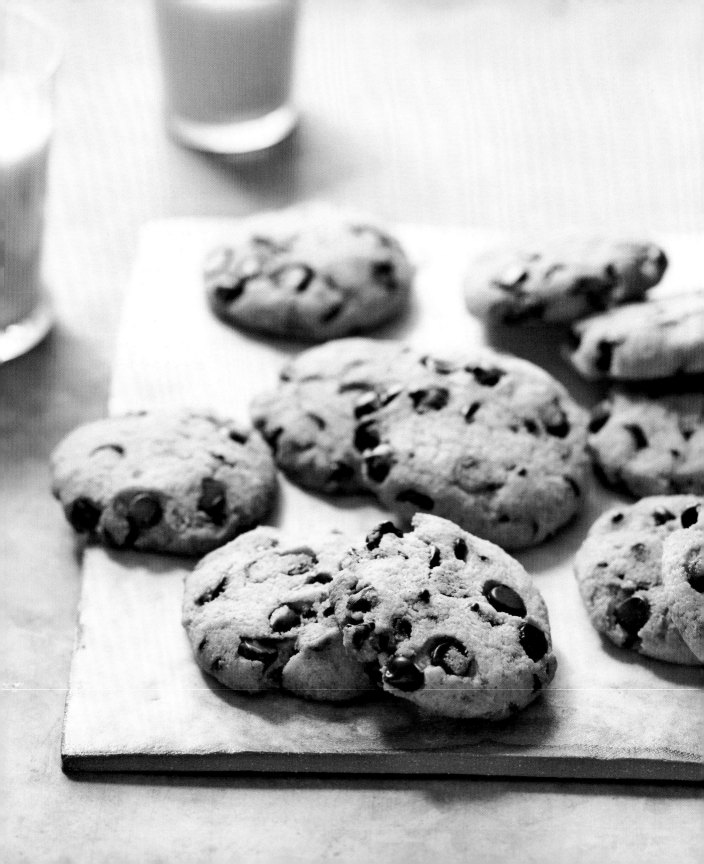

Once I discovered Lily's keto-friendly stevia-sweetened chocolate chips, I wanted to use them in everything. They taste amazing in these cookies.

CHOCOLATE CHIP COOKIES

PREHEAT the oven to 350°F. Line a baking sheet with parchment paper.

IN a large bowl, whisk together the melted butter, sweetener, stevia, eggs, and vanilla until combined.

IN a separate bowl, mix together the almond flour, coconut flour, baking powder, xanthan gum, and salt until combined. Add the dry ingredients to the wet ingredients and mix until fully incorporated. Using a spatula, gently fold in the chocolate chips until incorporated throughout.

USING your hands, roll about 1 tablespoon of dough into a ball, place on the prepared baking sheet, and flatten slightly. These cookies will not spread much when baked. Repeat with the remaining dough. Bake for 12 to 14 minutes, until golden brown. Let cool on the baking sheet for about 5 minutes before transferring them to a wire rack to cool completely.

KEEP cookies in an airtight container at room temperature for up to 5 days.

NUTRITIONAL INFO (PER SERVING)
CALORIES 79, **FAT** 7.3 g, **PROTEIN** 2.1 g, **CARBS** 5.6 g, **FIBER** 1.1 g

MAKES 24 SERVINGS

½ cup unsalted butter, melted

½ cup Swerve confectioners' sweetener

¼ cup Pyure powdered organic stevia (Bakeable Blend)

2 large eggs, whisked

1 teaspoon vanilla extract

1¼ cups blanched almond flour

¼ cup coconut flour

2 teaspoons baking powder

½ teaspoon xanthan gum

½ teaspoon pink Himalayan salt

1½ cups Lily's stevia-sweetened dark chocolate chips (one 9-ounce bag)

Look for peanut butter with no added sugar. I often use Smucker's natural peanut butter, which has nothing but nuts and salt.

THREE-INGREDIENT PEANUT BUTTER COOKIES

MAKES 15 SERVINGS

~~~

1 large egg

1 cup smooth peanut butter

½ cup monkfruit powdered sweetener

PREHEAT the oven to 350°F. Line a baking sheet with parchment paper or a silicone mat.

IN a bowl, mix together the egg, peanut butter, and sweetener until well combined.

USING your hands, roll 1 tablespoon of dough into a ball and place on the prepared baking sheet. Repeat with the rest of the dough. Using a fork, press down on the top of each ball in opposite directions to create a crisscross pattern.

BAKE for 12 to 15 minutes, until golden brown. Let cool on the baking sheet for about 5 minutes before transferring to a wire rack to cool completely. Keep cookies in an airtight container at room temperature for up to 5 days.

NUTRITIONAL INFO (PER SERVING)
CALORIES 108, **FAT** 9.2 g, **PROTEIN** 4.2 g, **CARBS** 6.5 g, **FIBER** 0.9 g

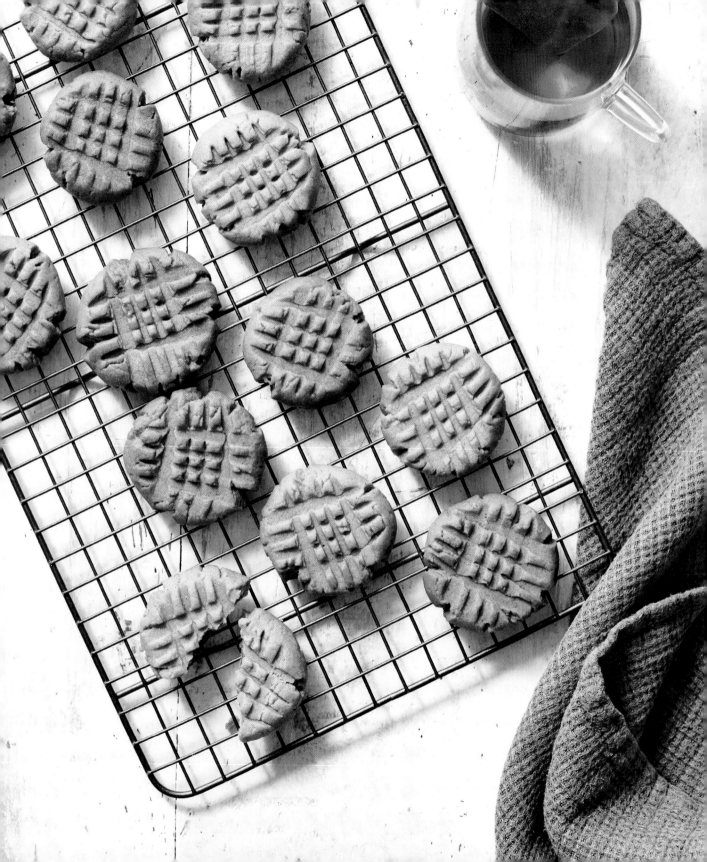

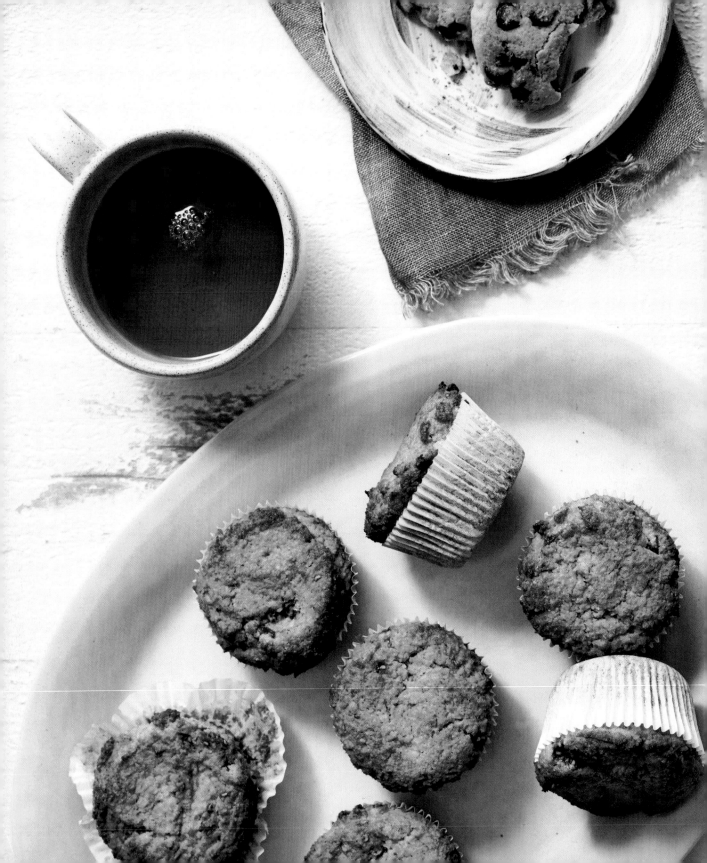

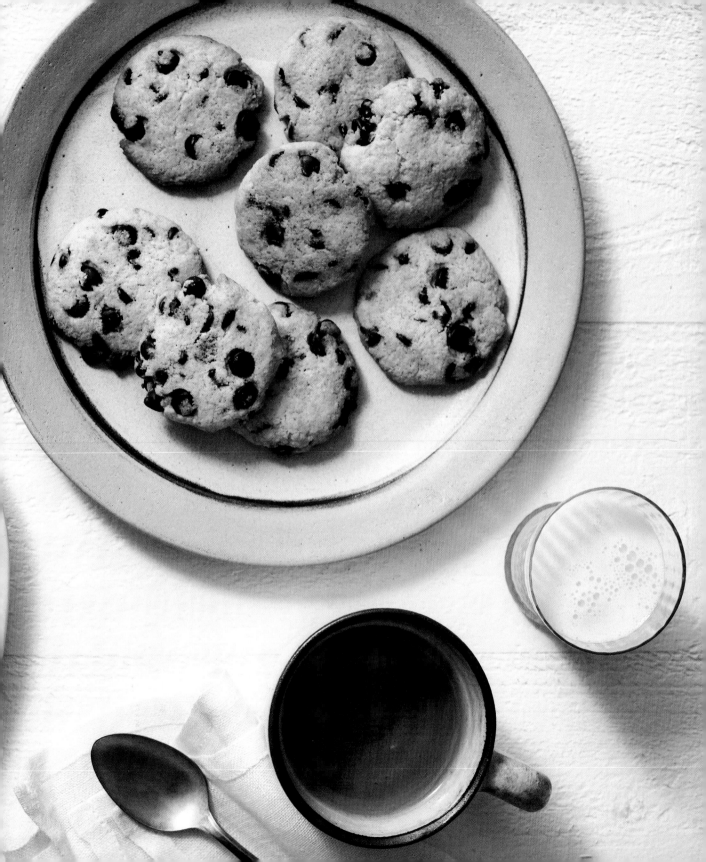

DRESSINGS, SEASONINGS & SAUCES

This is a delicious everyday salad dressing that also makes a nice marinade for beef, pork, and chicken.

BALSAMIC DRESSING AND MARINADE

IN a medium bowl, whisk together all the ingredients until emulsified. Store in a covered container in the refrigerator for up to 7 days.

NUTRITIONAL INFO (PER SERVING)
CALORIES 56, **FAT** 5.7 g, **PROTEIN** 0.2 g, **CARBS** 1.2 g, **FIBER** 0.2 g

**MAKES 1¼ CUPS
(20 SERVINGS)**

~~~

½ cup extra-virgin olive oil

¼ cup balsamic vinegar

3 tablespoons minced fresh parsley

2 tablespoons apple cider vinegar

2 tablespoons minced fresh basil

1 teaspoon grated lemon zest

1 tablespoon lemon juice

1 tablespoon Dijon mustard

1 tablespoon minced garlic

1 teaspoon dried oregano

½ teaspoon salt

¼ teaspoon black pepper

Use this creamy dressing on your favorite salad. The avocado amps up the healthy fat content you are looking for.

HOMEMADE AVOCADO CILANTRO DRESSING

COMBINE ½ cup water with all the ingredients in a food processor and pulse until smooth. Add more water if needed to reach your desired consistency. Store in a covered container in the refrigerator for up to 4 days.

NUTRITIONAL INFO (PER SERVING)
CALORIES 53, **FAT** 4.3 g, **PROTEIN** 1.4 g, **CARBS** 3.1 g, **FIBER** 1.2 g

**MAKES 2 CUPS
(16 SERVINGS)**

1 large avocado

1 cup fresh cilantro leaves

1 cup sour cream

1 teaspoon grated lime zest

1 tablespoon lime juice

1 teaspoon salt

½ teaspoon minced garlic

It's really easy to make pesto, so I make it myself instead of buying it.

BASIL PESTO

COMBINE the basil, Parmesan cheese, and walnuts in a food processor and pulse until chunky. Slowly drizzle in the olive oil and pulse to blend. Add the garlic, salt, and pepper and blend until it reaches a smooth consistency. Store in a covered container in the refrigerator for up to 5 to 7 days.

NUTRITIONAL INFO (PER SERVING)
CALORIES 98, **FAT** 10.3 g, **PROTEIN** 1.6 g, **CARBS** 0.4 g, **FIBER** 1.2 g

2 cups fresh basil leaves

⅔ cup grated Parmesan cheese

⅓ cup walnuts

½ cup extra-virgin olive oil

1 tablespoon minced garlic

1 teaspoon salt

½ teaspoon black pepper

Make mayonnaise from scratch and you'll never want to buy it again. It's that good.

HOMEMADE MAYO

COMBINE the egg, lemon zest and juice, vinegar, mustard, and salt in a food processor and process for about 30 seconds. With the motor running, add ½ cup of the avocado oil a few drops at a time. Go slow, this step should take 3 to 4 minutes. With the processor still running, gradually add the remaining ½ cup oil until the mayonnaise is thick. Store in a covered container in the refrigerator for up to 3 to 5 days.

1 large egg

1 teaspoon grated lemon zest

2 tablespoons lemon juice

1 teaspoon red wine vinegar

1 teaspoon Dijon mustard

½ teaspoon salt

1 cup avocado oil

NUTRITIONAL INFO (PER SERVING)
CALORIES 126, **FAT** 14 g, **PROTEIN** 0.4 g, **CARBS** 0.2 g, **FIBER** 0 g

I use this a lot, so I usually make a quadruple batch and keep some on hand.

HOMEMADE DRY RANCH SEASONING

COMBINE all the ingredients in a food processor and pulse until the mixture is roughly chopped. Store in a covered container at room temperature for up to 4 months.

NOTE: *To make a large batch to keep on hand, increase the amounts of ingredients as follows: ¼ cup dried parsley, 2 teaspoons garlic powder, 2 teaspoons dried dill, 1 teaspoon pink Himalayan salt, 1 teaspoon onion powder, and ½ teaspoon black pepper. This makes about 6 tablespoons seasoning.*

NUTRITIONAL INFO (PER SERVING)
CALORIES 20, **FAT** 0.2 g, **PROTEIN** 1.1 g, **CARBS** 4.5 g, **FIBER** 1.5 g

**MAKES ABOUT
1½ TABLESPOONS
(1 SERVING)**

1 tablespoon dried parsley

½ teaspoon garlic powder

½ teaspoon dried dill

¼ teaspoon pink Himalayan salt

¼ teaspoon onion powder

⅛ teaspoon black pepper

Kids really like ranch dressing so I wanted to be sure to include my recipe here.

HOMEMADE RANCH SALAD DRESSING

COMBINE all the ingredients in a blender and blend on high speed until smooth and creamy. Store in a covered container in the refrigerator for up to 5 to 7 days.

NUTRITIONAL INFO (PER SERVING)
CALORIES 51, **FAT** 4.9 g, **PROTEIN** 0.4 g, **CARBS** 1.2 g, **FIBER** 0.1 g

MAKES 1¾ CUPS (28 SERVINGS)

~~~

- ½ cup Homemade Mayo (page 229) or store-bought mayonnaise
- ½ cup sour cream
- ¼ cup lemon juice
- 2 tablespoons chopped fresh parsley
- 2 teaspoons onion powder
- 2 teaspoons dried dill
- 1 teaspoon garlic powder
- 1 teaspoon pink Himalayan salt
- ½ teaspoon black pepper

Homemade Avocado Cilantro Dressing, page 227

Homemade Salted Caramel Sauce, page 240

Hollandaise Sauce,
page 234

Homemade
No-Cook BBQ
Sauce, page 238

Homemade Marinara
Sauce, page 236

Use this for your eggs Benedict.

HOLLANDAISE SAUCE

USE a blender or an immersion blender to blend the egg yolks, lemon juice, salt, and cayenne together. Slowly add the melted butter and continue to blend. Season with black pepper, if using. Store in a covered container in the refrigerator for up to 1 day.

NUTRITIONAL INFO (PER SERVING)
CALORIES 73, **FAT** 4.8 g, **PROTEIN** 6.3 g, **CARBS** 0.9 g, **FIBER** 0 g

MAKES ⅓ CUP (2 SERVINGS)

2 large egg yolks

1 tablespoon lemon juice

⅛ teaspoon salt

Pinch cayenne pepper

8 tablespoons butter, melted

Black pepper, optional

It's always best to make your own taco seasoning because most of the store-bought brands contain sugar. The cocoa powder adds a depth of flavor without a prominent taste of chocolate. It's the secret ingredient!

TACO SEASONING

IN a small bowl, mix together all the ingredients. The seasoning keeps in an airtight container at room temperature for up to 12 months.

NOTE: *To make a large batch to keep on hand, increase the amounts of ingredients as follows: ¼ cup chili powder, 4 teaspoons unsweetened cocoa powder, 1 tablespoon ground cumin, 2 teaspoons salt, 2 teaspoons dried oregano, 1 teaspoon garlic powder, and 1 teaspoon onion powder. This makes about 6 tablespoons seasoning.*

NUTRITIONAL INFO (PER SERVING)
CALORIES 37, **FAT** 1.8 g, **PROTEIN** 2 g, **CARBS** 7.4 g, **FIBER** 4 g

**MAKES
2¼ TABLESPOONS
(2 SERVINGS)**

〰〰〰

1 tablespoon chili powder

1 teaspoon unsweetened cocoa powder

¾ teaspoon ground cumin

½ teaspoon salt

½ teaspoon dried oregano

¼ teaspoon garlic powder

¼ teaspoon onion powder

This is an amazingly versatile recipe. Use it in the lasagna (page 92), spaghetti squash (page 175), and calzone (page 95), or as a pizza sauce.

HOMEMADE MARINARA SAUCE

**MAKES 4 CUPS
(8 SERVINGS)**

IN a large pot, heat the olive oil over medium-low heat. Add the garlic and cook, stirring often to prevent burning, until it starts to turn light brown, 7 to 10 minutes. Add the tomatoes, stock, Parmesan, bay leaves, vinegar, basil, oregano, onion powder, salt, black pepper, and cayenne and stir to combine.

RAISE the heat, cover, and bring the ingredients to a low boil. Lower the heat to medium-low and simmer, stirring occasionally to make sure it doesn't stick to the bottom, until the flavors come together, 45 minutes to 1 hour.

DISCARD the bay leaves. Use immediately, or let the sauce cool completely and store in an airtight container in the refrigerator for up to 5 days or in the freezer for up to 4 months. To reheat, first let the sauce thaw at room temperature for about 1 hour, then reheat in the microwave or in a small saucepan on the stovetop.

NUTRITIONAL INFO (PER SERVING)
CALORIES 62, **FAT** 1.8 g, **PROTEIN** 3.4 g, **CARBS** 9.8 g, **FIBER** 2.3 g

1 teaspoon extra-virgin olive oil

1 tablespoon minced garlic

2 (28-ounce) cans crushed tomatoes

⅓ cup Stovetop Chicken Stock (page 67), vegetable stock, or store-bought broth

3 tablespoons grated Parmesan cheese

3 bay leaves

1 teaspoon apple cider vinegar

1½ teaspoons dried basil

1 teaspoon dried oregano

½ teaspoon onion powder

2 teaspoons salt

½ teaspoon black pepper

¼ teaspoon cayenne pepper

Store-bought ketchup almost always has sugar. The solution is to make it yourself!

HOMEMADE SUGAR-FREE KETCHUP

IN a blender, combine 2 tablespoons water with all the ingredients and blend on high until completely blended. Transfer to an airtight container and refrigerate for at least 1 hour before using. Ketchup keeps in an airtight container in the refrigerator for up to 2 weeks.

NUTRITIONAL INFO (PER SERVING)
CALORIES 16, **FAT** 0 g, **PROTEIN** 0.2 g, **CARBS** 4.1 g, **FIBER** 0.2 g

**MAKES ABOUT 1 CUP
(48 SERVINGS)**

6 ounces tomato paste

3 tablespoons apple cider vinegar

1 tablespoon Swerve brown sugar sweetener

2 teaspoons dry mustard

1½ teaspoons coconut aminos

¾ teaspoon pink Himalayan salt

½ teaspoon onion powder

¼ teaspoon ground allspice

¼ teaspoon black pepper

⅛ teaspoon cayenne pepper

Store-bought barbecue sauce almost always contains brown sugar or corn syrup. But that's no big deal because you can make your own and it's delicious!

NO-COOK BBQ SAUCE

MAKES 1 CUP (48 SERVINGS)

IN a small bowl, mix together all the ingredients and transfer to an airtight container. The sauce keeps in an airtight container in the refrigerator for up to 7 days.

NUTRITIONAL INFO (PER SERVING)
CALORIES 24, **FAT** 0.1 g, **PROTEIN** 0.1 g, **CARBS** 3.7 g, **FIBER** 3.8 g

1 cup Homemade Sugar-Free Ketchup (page 237) or store-bought sugar-free ketchup

2 tablespoons Frank's RedHot hot sauce

2 tablespoons Worcestershire sauce

1 tablespoon unsweetened cocoa powder

2 teaspoons dry mustard

2 teaspoons liquid smoke

2 teaspoons garlic powder

2 teaspoons ground cumin

1 teaspoon onion powder

1 teaspoon chili powder

1 teaspoon smoked paprika

This tastes so good. My advice? Make it and quickly pour it over veggies or cooked spaghetti squash for a quick meal.

HOMEMADE CHEESE SAUCE

IN a saucepan over medium heat, mix together all the ingredients and cook, stirring, until the cheese melts and the ingredients are fully combined. Lower the heat to medium-low and simmer, stirring, until the sauce thickens, 3 to 4 minutes. Let the sauce cool completely. It will thicken even more as it cools. Store in a covered container in the refrigerator for up to 1 week.

NUTRITIONAL INFO (PER SERVING)
CALORIES 119, **FAT** 11.5 g, **PROTEIN** 2.2 g, **CARBS** 2.2 g, **FIBER** 0 g

**MAKES 2 CUPS
(16 SERVINGS)**

1 cup heavy cream

4 ounces cream cheese

½ cup shredded cheddar cheese

¼ cup grated Parmesan cheese

3 tablespoons salted butter

2 teaspoons Frank's RedHot hot sauce

½ teaspoon garlic powder

¼ teaspoon dry mustard

¼ teaspoon salt

¼ teaspoon black pepper

Drizzle over Blueberry Pound Cake (page 214).

HOMEMADE SALTED CARAMEL SAUCE

IN a saucepan over medium heat, mix together the butter, yacon syrup, sweetener, and salt and bring to a boil, stirring frequently. Lower the heat to a simmer and slowly whisk in the cream. Be careful; the mixture will bubble up. Add the vanilla and xanthan gum, if using, and continue to cook, stirring, for another 2 minutes. Remove from the heat. The sauce will thicken as it cools. The caramel keeps in a covered container in the refrigerator for up to 1 week.

NUTRITIONAL INFO (PER SERVING)
CALORIES 233, **FAT** 25.4 g, **PROTEIN** 0.8 g, **CARBS** 4.7 g, **FIBER** 0 g

MAKES ¼ CUP (4 SERVINGS)

~~~~

6 tablespoons salted butter

2 teaspoons yacon syrup

2 teaspoons monkfruit golden sweetener

¼ teaspoon salt

6 tablespoons heavy cream

½ teaspoon vanilla extract

¾ teaspoon xanthan gum, optional (for thicker sauce)

This syrup is delicious and perfect when poured over Keto Pancakes (page 9) or Fluffy Keto Waffles (page 15).

HOMEMADE MAPLE SYRUP

IN a saucepan over medium heat, whisk together 1 cup water, the sweetener, maple extract, and vanilla and bring to a boil. Lower the heat and whisk in the xanthan gum. Remove from the heat. The syrup will thicken as it cools. Store in an airtight container at room temperature for up to 2 weeks.

NUTRITIONAL INFO (PER SERVING)
CALORIES 6, **FAT** 0 g, **PROTEIN** 0 g, **CARBS** 5.4 g, **FIBER** 0.1 g

**MAKES 1 CUP
(8 SERVINGS)**

½ cup monkfruit powdered sweetener

1 tablespoon maple extract

½ teaspoon vanilla extract

½ teaspoon xanthan gum

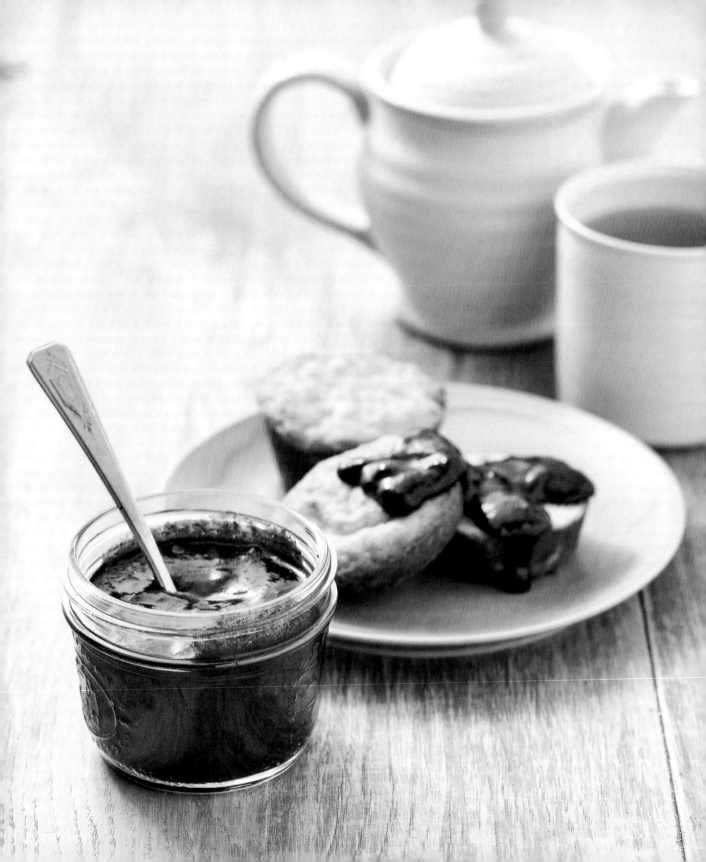

The flavor of Lakanto monkfruit sweetener is my personal favorite, but you can use stevia or erythritol. This sauce is the best on the Keto Pancakes (page 9).

BLUEBERRY SAUCE

IN a saucepan over low heat, combine ¼ cup water with the blueberries, sweetener, and lemon juice. Cook, stirring occasionally, until the fruit has reduced into a thick sauce, about 20 minutes. For a thicker sauce, smash the blueberries and stir frequently while cooking. If you like your sauce chunky, leave the blueberries whole while cooking, which will result in a compote. If you'd like to make the sauce a bit thicker, add the xanthan gum and stir thoroughly.

SERVE warm or let cool completely before storing. Store in a covered container in the refrigerator for up to 7 days. Reheat the sauce over low heat when you are ready to use it.

NUTRITIONAL INFO (PER SERVING)
CALORIES 13, **FAT** 0.1 g, **PROTEIN** 0.2 g, **CARBS** 3.9 g, **FIBER** 0.5 g

VARIATION
Replace the blueberries with chopped strawberries or raspberries and cook as directed.

**MAKES 1¼ CUPS
(20 SERVINGS)**

3 cups blueberries

3 tablespoons monkfruit powdered sweetener

2 tablespoons lemon juice

½ teaspoon xanthan gum, optional

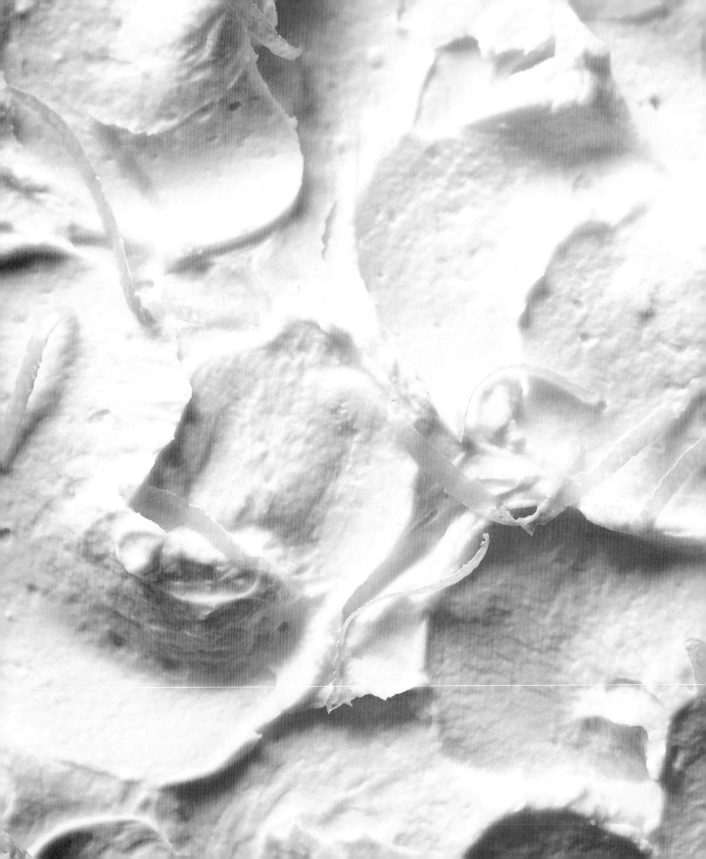

INDEX

Note: Page references in *italics* indicate photographs.

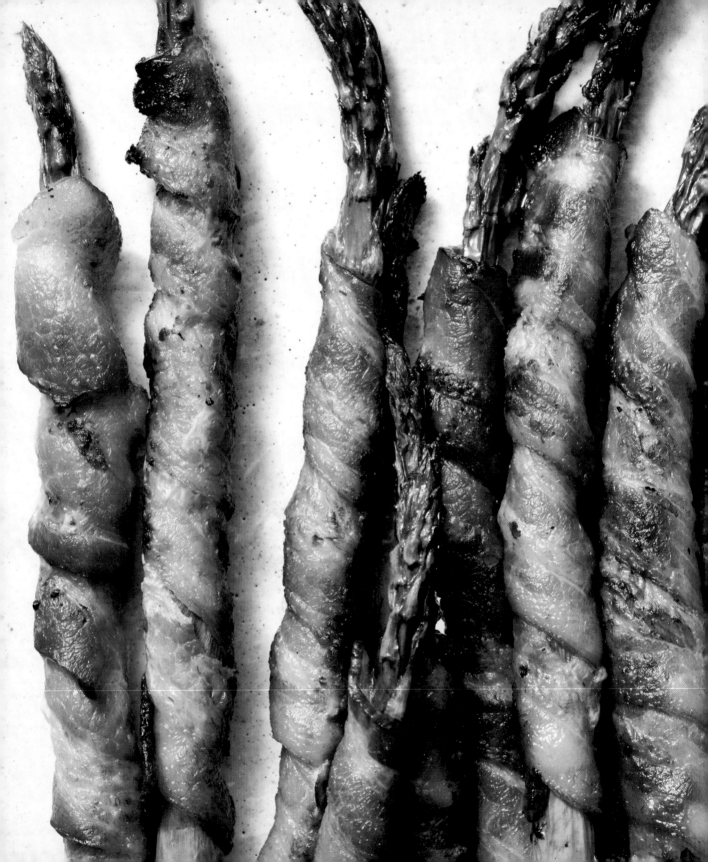